AYURVEDIC MANAGEMENT OF SKIN DISORDERS

Dr Mukesh Aggarwal

INDEX

PREFACE 5

PART 1 — Acne, Facial & Pigmentation Disorders 8

1. Acne Vulgaris (Yuvan Pidika) 9
2. Teenage, Adult & Hormonal Acne 14
3. Cystic Acne, Acne Scars & Post-Acne Care 20
4. Blackheads, Whiteheads & Open Pores 26
5. Oily, Dry, Sensitive & Combination Skin Disorders 32
6. Hyperpigmentation & Facial Pigmentation 38
7. Melasma & Post-Inflammatory Hyperpigmentation 44
8. Dark Circles, Facial Dullness & Loss of Glow 50
9. Facial Redness, Rosacea & Flushing Disorder 55

PART 2 — Chronic Inflammatory & Autoimmune Skin Disorders 61

10. Eczema (Vicharchika) & Atopic Dermatitis 62
11. Contact & Seborrheic Dermatitis 68
12. Psoriasis (Kitibha Kushta) 74
13. Vitiligo (Shwitra) 80
14. Urticaria (Sheetapitta) & Allergic Skin Disorders 85
15. Chronic Pruritus & Xerotic Skin Disorders 90
16. Autoimmune & Immune Dysregulation 96
17. Reactive Sensitive Skin & Chronic Facial Inflammation 102
18. Recurrent Eczema, Psoriasis & Allergic Dermatoses 108

PART 3 — Infectious Skin Disorders 114

19. Fungal Skin Infections & Dermatophytosis 115
20. Tinea Pedis, Intertrigo & Recurrent Fungal Disorders 120
21. Bacterial Skin Infections, Furunculosis & Carbuncles 125
22. Folliculitis, Abscesses & Recurrent Boils 130
23. Viral Skin Disorders 135

24. Nail Disorders & Fungal Nail Infections 140

PART 4 — Cosmetic, Aging & Aesthetic Dermatology 146

25. Cosmetic-Induced Dermatitis & Steroid 147
26. Premature Aging, Wrinkles & Senile Skin Changes 153
27. Sun-Damaged Skin & Photoaging 159
28. Menopausal & Age-Related Skin Disorders 164
29. Skin Barrier Dysfunction & Dehydrated 170
30. Facial Puffiness, Roughness & Enlarged Pores 176
31. Skin Tags & Benign Cosmetic Skin Disorders 181
32. Integrative Ayurvedic Cosmeto-Dermatology 187

PART 5 — Lifestyle, Hormonal & Systemic Skin Disorders 193

33. Hormonal & PCOS-Associated Skin Disorders 194
34. Digestive-Origin & Constipation-Associated 200
35. Nutritional Deficiency & Metabolic Toxicity 206
36. Stress, Anxiety & Sleep-Deprivation Related 212
37. Urban Pollution, Smoking & Environmental Toxicity 218
38. Seasonal Skin Disorders, Heat Rashes & Prickly Heat 224
39. Occupational, Hard Water & Digital Lifestyle 230
40. Chronic Wound Healing, Low Immunity & Neuro-Endocrine Skin Disorders 236

PART 6 — Dosha-Based Dermatology 242

41. Vataja Skin Disorders 243
42. Pittaja Skin Disorders 249
43. Kaphaja Skin Disorders 255

BIBLIOGRAPHY 261

PREFACE

Skin is not merely the outer covering of the body; it is a reflection of internal health, emotional balance, nutrition, immunity, hormonal harmony, and overall wellbeing. In Ayurveda, healthy skin is considered a sign of balanced Doshas, proper digestion, pure Rakta Dhatu, strong immunity, and a peaceful mind. When these internal systems become disturbed, the skin often becomes the first organ to express imbalance through acne, pigmentation, allergies, eczema, psoriasis, premature aging, infections, and numerous other dermatological conditions.

In modern times, the prevalence of skin disorders has increased tremendously due to stress, pollution, unhealthy diet, hormonal imbalance, sedentary lifestyle, excessive cosmetic use, disturbed sleep, and environmental toxicity. While conventional dermatology offers symptomatic relief in many cases, Ayurveda provides a holistic and root-cause-oriented approach by correcting internal imbalance, detoxifying the body, improving immunity, and rejuvenating skin health naturally.

This book, *Ayurvedic Management of Skin Disorders*, has been written with the aim of integrating classical Ayurvedic wisdom with practical clinical understanding of modern dermatological conditions. Every chapter has been designed in a concise and clinically useful format including:

- Introduction of the disorder
- Classical Ayurvedic references and Sanskrit shlokas
- Nidana (causes)
- Samprapti (pathogenesis)
- Lakshana (symptoms)
- Ayurvedic management

- Classical medicines with dosage, Anupana, and duration
- Panchakarma therapies
- Pathya-Apathya (diet and lifestyle)
- Prognosis and conclusion

Special emphasis has been given to common contemporary skin disorders including acne, pigmentation, fungal infections, psoriasis, eczema, hormonal skin disorders, cosmetic dermatology, anti-aging care, pollution-induced damage, stress-related skin disorders, and integrative cosmeto-dermatology.

The purpose of this book is not only to provide therapeutic guidance but also to encourage preventive skin care through proper lifestyle, mental wellbeing, balanced nutrition, detoxification, and Ayurvedic daily regimens. Ayurveda teaches us that true beauty arises from internal harmony, purity, and vitality.

I sincerely hope this book will serve as a valuable guide for Ayurvedic physicians, dermatologists, students, cosmetologists, healthcare professionals, and all readers interested in holistic skin care and natural healing.

With gratitude to the great Ayurvedic Acharyas whose timeless wisdom continues to illuminate the path of healing.

Dr. Mukesh Aggarwal
Founder & Managing Director
VHCA HAIR & SKIN CLINIC

PART 1

ACNE, FACIAL & PIGMENTATION DISORDERS

Chapter 1

ACNE VULGARIS (YUVAN PIDIKA)

Introduction

In Ayurveda, acne is described under **Yuvan Pidika** or **Mukhadushika**, commonly occurring during adolescence due to vitiation of Kapha, Vata, and Rakta along with Meda Dushti. The eruptions resemble the thorns of the Shalmali tree and mainly appear on the face, causing inflammation, pain, discoloration, and scarring.

Classical Reference (श्लोक)

"मुखे यौवनपीडिकाः शाल्मलीकण्टकोपमाः ।
कफवातसमुत्थानाः मेदोरक्तप्रदूषिताः ॥"

— Sushruta Samhita

Meaning

During youth, eruptions resembling thorns of the silk cotton tree appear on the face due to vitiation of Kapha and Vata along with impurity of Rakta and Meda.

Another reference:

"युवानां मुखदूषिकाः पिडिकाः स्युः विशेषतः।"

Meaning: Facial eruptions commonly occurring in youth are termed Mukhadushika.

Nidana (Causes)

- Excess oily, spicy, fried food
- Excess sweets and junk food

- Hormonal imbalance
- Stress and anxiety
- Irregular sleep
- Constipation and poor digestion
- Excessive cosmetics and chemical exposure
- Suppression of natural urges
- Excess sweating and pollution

Samprapti (Pathogenesis)

Aggravated Kapha and Pitta vitiate Rakta and Meda Dhatu. The vitiated Doshas localize in facial skin and block hair follicles and sweat channels, producing inflammatory eruptions. Vata contributes to pain and scarring.

Lakshana (Symptoms)

- Pimples and pustules on face
- Oily skin
- Redness and inflammation
- Pain or tenderness
- Blackheads and whiteheads
- Acne scars and pigmentation
- Burning or itching sensation

Ayurvedic Management

1. Shamana Chikitsa (Internal Medicines)

Gandhak Rasayan

Dosage: 250–500 mg twice daily
Anupana: Honey or lukewarm water
Duration: 2–3 months

Kaishore Guggulu

Dosage: 1–2 tablets twice daily
Anupana: Warm water
Duration: 2–4 months

Mahamanjishthadi Kwath

Dosage: 15–20 ml twice daily after meals
Anupana: Equal quantity of water
Duration: 3 months

Arogyavardhini Vati

Dosage: 250 mg twice daily
Anupana: Lukewarm water
Duration: 2 months

Avipattikar Churna

(Useful in Pitta-dominant acne with constipation)

Dosage: 3–5 grams at bedtime
Anupana: Lukewarm water
Duration: 1–2 months

2. External Therapies

Lepa (Herbal Face Packs)

Recommended Herbs

- Lodhra
- Neem
- Turmeric
- Manjistha
- Rakta Chandan

Apply paste once daily for 20–30 minutes.

Neem Taila Application

Useful in infected and inflammatory acne lesions.

Steam with Neem Decoction

Helps in cleansing pores and reducing oiliness.

3. Panchakarma

Virechana

Best therapy in Pitta-Rakta dominant acne.

Raktamokshana

Useful in severe inflammatory and recurrent acne.

Nasya

Helps in facial skin purification and hormonal balance.

Pathya (Wholesome Diet & Lifestyle)

Recommended Foods

- Amla
- Neem preparations
- Green vegetables
- Bottle gourd
- Mung dal
- Pomegranate
- Coconut water
- Buttermilk
- Warm water

Healthy Practices

- Adequate sleep
- Daily facial cleansing
- Yoga and meditation
- Stress reduction
- Regular bowel habits
- Use of herbal skin cleansers

Apathya (To Avoid)

- Excess spicy, sour, salty foods
- Fried and junk foods
- Excess chocolates and bakery items
- Carbonated drinks
- Late-night sleeping
- Excess cosmetics
- Picking or squeezing pimples
- Smoking and alcohol

Prognosis (Sadhya-Asadhyata)

- Mild and recent acne: Generally Sadhya (curable)
- Chronic cystic acne with scarring: Yapya (manageable)
- Early treatment helps prevent scars and pigmentation.

Conclusion

Yuvan Pidika is primarily a disorder of Kapha, Pitta, Rakta, and Meda Dushti affecting facial skin during adolescence and hormonal imbalance. Ayurveda offers holistic management through purification therapies, blood purification, herbal medicines, dietary correction, and lifestyle regulation.

Chapter 2

TEENAGE, ADULT & HORMONAL ACNE

Introduction

Teenage, adult, and hormonal acne are chronic inflammatory disorders of the pilosebaceous units characterized by pimples, pustules, nodules, excessive oiliness, and recurrent breakouts. In Ayurveda, these conditions are considered variations of **Yuvan Pidika** and arise due to vitiation of Kapha, Pitta, Rakta, and Meda. Hormonal disturbances, stress, improper diet, and impaired digestion play major roles in recurrent acne.

Classical Reference (श्लोक)

"मुखदूषिका नाम कफवातप्रकोपजा ।
मेदोरक्तसमुद्भूता यौवने विशेषतः ॥"

— Ayurvedic Classical Reference

Meaning

Mukhadushika arises due to aggravated Kapha and Vata along with vitiation of Meda and Rakta, especially during youth.

Another reference:

"पित्तं रक्तं च दूष्येते मुखे पिडिकाः भवन्ति।"

Meaning: Vitiation of Pitta and Rakta leads to eruptions on the face.

Nidana (Causes)

- Pubertal hormonal changes
- PCOS and endocrine imbalance
- Excess oily and spicy food
- Stress, anxiety, anger
- Poor digestion and constipation
- Excess cosmetics and steroid creams
- Irregular sleep
- Menstrual irregularities
- Excess sugar and dairy intake
- Sedentary lifestyle

Samprapti (Pathogenesis)

Aggravated Pitta and Kapha vitiate Rakta and Meda Dhatu. Increased oil secretion blocks skin pores and causes inflammation. Hormonal imbalance further aggravates Meda and Kapha, while Vata contributes to recurrent eruptions and scarring.

Lakshana (Symptoms)

- Recurrent pimples
- Painful cystic eruptions
- Oily skin
- Acne before menstruation
- Pigmentation and scars
- Blackheads and whiteheads
- Facial redness and inflammation
- Irregular menstrual cycle in females

Ayurvedic Management

1. Shamana Chikitsa (Internal Medicines)

Kaishore Guggulu

Dosage: 1–2 tablets twice daily
Anupana: Warm water
Duration: 2–4 months

Gandhak Rasayan

Dosage: 250–500 mg twice daily
Anupana: Honey
Duration: 3 months

Mahamanjishthadi Kwath

Dosage: 15–20 ml twice daily after meals
Anupana: Equal quantity of water
Duration: 3 months

Kumaryasava

(Useful in hormonal imbalance and PCOS-associated acne)

Dosage: 15–20 ml twice daily
Anupana: Equal quantity of water
Duration: 2–3 months

Avipattikar Churna

Dosage: 3–5 grams at bedtime
Anupana: Warm water
Duration: 1–2 months

2. External Therapies

Mukhalepa

Herbal paste of:

- Neem
- Lodhra
- Turmeric
- Manjistha
- Rakta Chandan

Apply once daily for 20–30 minutes.

Steam Therapy

Neem or Triphala steam helps open pores and reduce oiliness.

Herbal Cleansing

Use mild herbal cleansers containing neem or aloe vera.

3. Panchakarma

Virechana

Best for Pitta-dominant inflammatory acne.

Raktamokshana

Useful in severe recurrent acne and pigmentation.

Nasya

Helps improve facial skin health and hormonal regulation.

Pathya (Wholesome Diet & Lifestyle)

Recommended Foods

- Amla
- Neem
- Green leafy vegetables
- Mung dal
- Pomegranate
- Coconut water
- Bitter vegetables
- Buttermilk
- Warm water

Healthy Practices

- Adequate sleep
- Daily exercise
- Yoga and meditation
- Stress management
- Regular bowel habits
- Gentle skin cleansing

Apathya (To Avoid)

- Fried and junk foods
- Excess spicy and sour foods
- Ice cream and excess dairy
- Excess sugar and bakery items
- Late-night sleeping
- Picking acne lesions
- Excess makeup and steroid creams
- Smoking and alcohol

Prognosis (Sadhya-Asadhyata)

- Mild teenage acne: Sadhya (curable)

- Hormonal and recurrent adult acne: Yapya (manageable)
- Early treatment prevents deep scars and pigmentation.

Conclusion

Teenage, adult, and hormonal acne reflect internal Dosha imbalance involving Kapha, Pitta, Rakta, and Meda. Ayurveda treats the root cause through blood purification, digestive correction, hormonal balance, Panchakarma, and lifestyle regulation. Proper Ayurvedic management helps control inflammation, reduce recurrence, and improve overall skin health naturally.

Chapter 3

CYSTIC ACNE, ACNE SCARS & POST-ACNE CARE

Introduction

Cystic acne is a severe inflammatory form of acne characterized by deep painful nodules, cysts, pus-filled lesions, and permanent scarring. In Ayurveda, it is considered an advanced stage of **Yuvan Pidika** involving profound vitiation of Pitta, Kapha, Rakta, and Meda along with obstruction of skin channels. Improper healing often results in scars, pigmentation, and uneven skin texture.

Classical Reference (श्लोक)

"कफवातसमुत्थानाः पिडिकाः शाल्मलीसमाः ।
रक्तमेदोदुष्टिजन्याः शोफदाहसमन्विताः ॥"

— Ayurvedic Classical Reference

Meaning

Skin eruptions arising from vitiated Kapha and Vata associated with impure Rakta and Meda produce swelling, inflammation, and painful lesions.

Another reference:

"दूषितं रक्तमाश्रित्य पित्तं दाहं प्रजायते।"

Meaning: Vitiated Pitta affecting Rakta produces inflammation and tissue damage.

Nidana (Causes)

- Untreated chronic acne
- Hormonal imbalance
- Excess oily and spicy food
- Excessive stress and anxiety
- Picking and squeezing pimples
- Poor digestion and constipation
- Excess cosmetic products
- Sleep deprivation
- Excess heat exposure
- Genetic predisposition

Samprapti (Pathogenesis)

Aggravated Pitta and Rakta produce intense inflammation in skin tissues. Kapha causes pus formation and cystic swelling, while Vata leads to tissue destruction and scar formation. Obstruction of microchannels impairs healing and causes pigmentation and fibrosis.

Lakshana (Symptoms)

- Painful cystic eruptions
- Deep nodules and abscess-like lesions
- Pus discharge
- Facial swelling and redness
- Acne scars and pits
- Dark pigmentation after healing
- Burning and tenderness
- Uneven skin texture

Ayurvedic Management

1. Shamana Chikitsa (Internal Medicines)

Kaishore Guggulu

Dosage: 1–2 tablets twice daily
Anupana: Warm water
Duration: 3–4 months

Gandhak Rasayan

Dosage: 250–500 mg twice daily
Anupana: Honey
Duration: 3 months

Mahamanjishthadi Kwath

Dosage: 15–20 ml twice daily
Anupana: Equal quantity of water
Duration: 3 months

Khadirarishta

Dosage: 15–20 ml twice daily after meals
Anupana: Equal quantity of water
Duration: 2–3 months

Avipattikar Churna

Dosage: 3–5 grams at bedtime
Anupana: Warm water
Duration: 1–2 months

2. External Therapies

Mukhalepa (Face Pack)

Ingredients:

- Manjistha
- Lodhra
- Neem
- Turmeric
- Rakta Chandan

Apply daily for 20–30 minutes.

Jatyadi Taila

Useful in healing acne scars and damaged skin.

Aloe Vera Gel Application

Helps soothe inflammation and improve healing.

3. Panchakarma

Virechana

Best for severe Pitta-Rakta dominant cystic acne.

Raktamokshana

Highly beneficial in recurrent inflammatory acne.

Vamana

Useful in Kapha-dominant oily cystic acne.

Pathya (Wholesome Diet & Lifestyle)

Recommended Foods

- Amla
- Neem
- Green vegetables

- Bitter gourd
- Pomegranate
- Coconut water
- Mung dal
- Buttermilk
- Fresh fruits

Healthy Practices

- Proper facial hygiene
- Stress management
- Adequate hydration
- Yoga and meditation
- Regular bowel habits
- Avoid touching lesions

Apathya (To Avoid)

- Fried and oily foods
- Excess sweets and dairy
- Spicy and sour foods
- Picking acne lesions
- Excess cosmetics
- Smoking and alcohol
- Late-night sleeping
- Excess heat and sun exposure

Prognosis (Sadhya-Asadhyata)

- Mild cystic acne: Krichra Sadhya (difficult but curable)
- Deep scarring acne: Yapya (manageable)
- Early intervention prevents permanent scarring and pigmentation.

Conclusion

Cystic acne and acne scars represent deeper involvement of Pitta, Rakta, Kapha, and Meda causing chronic inflammation and tissue damage. Ayurveda offers holistic management through blood purification, anti-inflammatory herbs, Panchakarma, healing therapies, and dietary correction. Timely Ayurvedic care helps reduce cyst formation, minimize scars, and restore healthy skin naturally.

Chapter 4

BLACKHEADS, WHITEHEADS & OPEN PORES

Introduction

Blackheads, whiteheads, and enlarged open pores are common cosmetic skin disorders associated with excessive oil secretion, blockage of skin channels, and accumulation of impurities within hair follicles. In Ayurveda, these conditions are related to vitiation of Kapha, Vata, and Meda along with obstruction of **Srotas** (microchannels). Improper cleansing, poor digestion, hormonal imbalance, and excess oily foods contribute to their development.

Classical Reference (श्लोक)

"कफमेदोवृताः स्रोतांसि त्वचि दोषान् प्रकोपयेत् ।
ततः पिडिकाः सूक्ष्माश्च मुखदूषिकाः प्रजायते ॥"

— Ayurvedic Classical Reference

Meaning

When Kapha and Meda obstruct skin channels, small eruptions and facial skin disorders develop.

Another reference:

"मेदोदुष्ट्या त्वचि स्निग्धता अधिका भवति।"

Meaning: Vitiation of Meda causes excessive oiliness of the skin.

Nidana (Causes)

- Excess oily and fried food
- Poor facial hygiene
- Hormonal imbalance
- Excessive cosmetic use
- Pollution and dust exposure
- Constipation and indigestion
- Excess sweating
- Stress and irregular sleep
- Sedentary lifestyle

Samprapti (Pathogenesis)

Aggravated Kapha and Meda increase oil secretion and clog skin pores. Accumulated impurities block follicles leading to formation of whiteheads and blackheads. Vata causes roughness and enlargement of pores, while Pitta may produce inflammation.

Lakshana (Symptoms)

- Blackheads on nose and face
- Whiteheads and tiny bumps
- Enlarged skin pores
- Oily and greasy skin
- Rough skin texture
- Mild inflammation
- Dull complexion

Ayurvedic Management

1. Shamana Chikitsa (Internal Medicines)

Arogyavardhini Vati

Dosage: 250 mg twice daily
Anupana: Lukewarm water
Duration: 2 months

Kaishore Guggulu

Dosage: 1 tablet twice daily
Anupana: Warm water
Duration: 2–3 months

Triphala Churna

Dosage: 3–5 grams at bedtime
Anupana: Warm water
Duration: 2 months

Gandhak Rasayan

Dosage: 250 mg twice daily
Anupana: Honey
Duration: 2 months

2. External Therapies

Herbal Face Pack (Mukhalepa)

Ingredients:

- Lodhra
- Neem
- Multani Mitti
- Turmeric
- Manjistha

Apply 3–4 times weekly for 20 minutes.

Steam Therapy

Steam with neem or Triphala decoction helps unclog pores.

Herbal Scrubbing

Gentle exfoliation using herbal powders helps remove dead skin and impurities.

Rose Water Cleansing

Useful in tightening pores and refreshing skin.

3. Panchakarma

Virechana

Useful in Pitta-Kapha dominant oily skin disorders.

Nasya

Helps improve facial circulation and skin clarity.

Raktamokshana

Indicated in recurrent inflammatory lesions.

Pathya (Wholesome Diet & Lifestyle)

Recommended Foods

- Green vegetables
- Amla
- Pomegranate
- Mung dal
- Buttermilk

- Coconut water
- Warm water
- Bitter vegetables

Healthy Practices

- Regular facial cleansing
- Adequate hydration
- Yoga and exercise
- Proper sleep
- Stress reduction
- Use non-comedogenic herbal products

Apathya (To Avoid)

- Oily and fried food
- Excess sweets and dairy
- Heavy cosmetics
- Excess touching of face
- Late-night sleeping
- Smoking and alcohol
- Excessive junk food
- Harsh chemical scrubs

Prognosis (Sadhya-Asadhyata)

- Mild blackheads and whiteheads: Sadhya (curable)
- Chronic enlarged pores with oily skin: Yapya (manageable)
- Early skin care prevents acne progression and scarring.

Conclusion

Blackheads, whiteheads, and open pores result from Kapha-Meda imbalance and blockage of skin channels. Ayurveda emphasizes purification, digestive correction, herbal cleansing, and healthy lifestyle practices to restore skin balance naturally. Regular Ayurvedic care helps maintain clear, smooth, and healthy skin while preventing recurrence.

Chapter 5

OILY, DRY, SENSITIVE & COMBINATION SKIN DISORDERS

Introduction

Skin type disorders such as oily, dry, sensitive, and combination skin occur due to imbalance of Doshas affecting the skin and its natural barrier. In Ayurveda, skin health depends upon the balance of Vata, Pitta, Kapha, Rakta, and proper nourishment of Rasa Dhatu. Vata predominance leads to dryness, Kapha causes excessive oiliness, while Pitta aggravation produces sensitivity, redness, and irritation.

Classical Reference (श्लोक)

"त्वचा रससमुत्पन्ना दोषैर्दूष्यति सर्वदा ।
वातात् शुष्कता ज्ञेया पित्ताद्दाहः कफात्स्निग्धता ॥"

— Ayurvedic Classical Reference

Meaning

Skin originates from Rasa Dhatu and becomes affected by Doshas. Vata causes dryness, Pitta causes burning and sensitivity, while Kapha produces oiliness.

Another reference:

"रक्तपित्तप्रकोपेन त्वचि दाहो विकारकृत्।"

Meaning: Aggravated Pitta and Rakta produce irritation and inflammatory skin changes.

Nidana (Causes)

- Improper diet and lifestyle
- Excess spicy, oily, or dry food
- Excess cosmetic and chemical exposure
- Stress and sleep deprivation
- Environmental pollution
- Hard water exposure
- Dehydration
- Excess sun exposure
- Seasonal changes
- Hormonal imbalance

Samprapti (Pathogenesis)

Aggravated Doshas affect skin channels and disturb natural moisture and oil balance. Vata reduces hydration causing dryness and roughness, Kapha increases sebum production leading to oily skin, while Pitta causes inflammation, redness, and hypersensitivity.

Lakshana (Symptoms)

Oily Skin

- Excess sebum
- Sticky skin
- Enlarged pores
- Acne tendency

Dry Skin

- Roughness

- Flaking
- Tightness
- Itching

Sensitive Skin

- Burning sensation
- Redness
- Irritation
- Allergy tendency

Combination Skin

- Oily T-zone
- Dry cheeks
- Uneven texture

Ayurvedic Management

1. Shamana Chikitsa (Internal Medicines)

Mahatikta Ghrita

(Useful in sensitive and inflammatory skin)

Dosage: 5–10 grams daily
Anupana: Lukewarm water or milk
Duration: 2–3 months

Gandhak Rasayan

Dosage: 250 mg twice daily
Anupana: Honey
Duration: 2 months

Sarivadyasava

Dosage: 15–20 ml twice daily
Anupana: Equal quantity of water
Duration: 2–3 months

Avipattikar Churna

(For Pitta-related sensitivity)

Dosage: 3–5 grams at bedtime
Anupana: Warm water
Duration: 1–2 months

2. External Therapies

For Oily Skin

- Neem and Multani Mitti face pack
- Gentle herbal cleansing

For Dry Skin

- Kumkumadi Taila massage
- Aloe vera and sandalwood application

For Sensitive Skin

- Rose water compress
- Chandan and Yashtimadhu paste

For Combination Skin

- Mild herbal cleansing with balanced moisturization

3. Panchakarma

Virechana

Best for Pitta-related sensitive skin disorders.

Nasya

Improves facial nourishment and skin texture.

Abhyanga

Useful in dry and Vata-dominant skin disorders.

Pathya (Wholesome Diet & Lifestyle)

Recommended Foods

- Amla
- Cow's ghee
- Coconut water
- Green vegetables
- Fresh fruits
- Soaked almonds
- Mung dal
- Buttermilk

Healthy Practices

- Adequate hydration
- Regular sleep
- Stress reduction
- Gentle skincare routine
- Daily oil massage
- Yoga and meditation

Apathya (To Avoid)

- Harsh chemical cosmetics
- Excess spicy and fried foods
- Over-cleansing of skin
- Smoking and alcohol
- Excess sun exposure
- Late-night sleeping
- Excess tea and coffee

Prognosis (Sadhya-Asadhyata)

- Mild skin imbalance: Sadhya (curable)
- Chronic sensitive skin disorders: Yapya (manageable)
- Early correction prevents premature aging and chronic inflammation.

Conclusion

Oily, dry, sensitive, and combination skin disorders reflect underlying Dosha imbalance and impaired skin nourishment. Ayurveda offers individualized management through Dosha correction, herbal medicines, Panchakarma, proper skincare, diet, and lifestyle regulation. Holistic Ayurvedic care helps restore natural skin balance, glow, hydration, and resilience naturally.

Chapter 6

HYPERPIGMENTATION & FACIAL PIGMENTATION

Introduction

Hyperpigmentation and facial pigmentation are common skin disorders characterized by dark patches, uneven skin tone, and discoloration due to excess melanin deposition. In Ayurveda, these conditions are associated with vitiation of Pitta, Rakta, and Bhrajaka Pitta affecting the skin complexion. Excess sun exposure, hormonal imbalance, inflammation, stress, and improper diet commonly aggravate pigmentation disorders.

Classical Reference (श्लोक)

"पित्ताद्रक्तप्रदुष्टत्वात् त्वचो वर्णविपर्ययः ।
श्यावता दाहयुक्ता च त्वग्विकाराः प्रजायते ॥"

— Ayurvedic Classical Reference

Meaning

Vitiation of Pitta and Rakta causes discoloration and abnormal pigmentation of the skin associated with burning sensation.

Another reference:

"भ्राजकपित्तदुष्ट्या त्वचि वर्णभेदो भवति।"

Meaning: Disturbance of Bhrajaka Pitta leads to changes in skin complexion and pigmentation.

Nidana (Causes)

- Excess sunlight exposure
- Hormonal imbalance
- Acne and inflammatory skin disorders
- Stress and anxiety
- Excess spicy and sour food
- Chemical cosmetics
- Pregnancy-related pigmentation
- Lack of sleep
- Nutritional deficiency
- Chronic digestive disturbances

Samprapti (Pathogenesis)

Aggravated Pitta and Rakta affect Bhrajaka Pitta in the skin, leading to abnormal melanin deposition and discoloration. Vata contributes to uneven texture while Kapha may cause dullness and thickening of skin.

Lakshana (Symptoms)

- Dark facial patches
- Uneven skin tone
- Brown or black discoloration
- Dull complexion
- Pigmentation after acne
- Sun-induced darkening
- Dryness or mild irritation

Ayurvedic Management

1. Shamana Chikitsa (Internal Medicines)

Mahamanjishthadi Kwath

Dosage: 15–20 ml twice daily after meals
Anupana: Equal quantity of water
Duration: 3 months

Khadirarishta

Dosage: 15–20 ml twice daily
Anupana: Equal quantity of water
Duration: 2–3 months

Gandhak Rasayan

Dosage: 250 mg twice daily
Anupana: Honey
Duration: 2 months

Arogyavardhini Vati

Dosage: 250 mg twice daily
Anupana: Lukewarm water
Duration: 2 months

Avipattikar Churna

Dosage: 3–5 grams at bedtime
Anupana: Warm water
Duration: 1–2 months

2. External Therapies

Mukhalepa (Face Pack)

Ingredients:

- Manjistha
- Lodhra
- Sandalwood
- Turmeric
- Yashtimadhu

Apply daily or alternate days for 20–30 minutes.

Kumkumadi Taila

Gentle facial massage at night helps improve complexion and reduce pigmentation.

Aloe Vera Application

Useful in soothing skin and reducing sun damage.

3. Panchakarma

Virechana

Best therapy for Pitta-Rakta dominant pigmentation disorders.

Raktamokshana

Useful in stubborn and recurrent pigmentation.

Nasya

Improves facial complexion and nourishment.

Pathya (Wholesome Diet & Lifestyle)

Recommended Foods

- Amla
- Pomegranate
- Coconut water
- Green vegetables

- Cow's ghee
- Fresh fruits
- Mung dal
- Bitter vegetables

Healthy Practices

- Use natural sun protection
- Adequate hydration
- Proper sleep
- Stress management
- Gentle skincare routine
- Yoga and meditation

Apathya (To Avoid)

- Excess sunlight exposure
- Spicy, sour, and fried foods
- Excess tea and coffee
- Harsh cosmetics and bleaching agents
- Smoking and alcohol
- Late-night sleeping
- Excess stress and anger

Prognosis (Sadhya-Asadhyata)

- Recent and mild pigmentation: Sadhya (curable)
- Chronic deep pigmentation: Yapya (manageable)
- Early treatment gives better improvement in complexion.

Conclusion

Hyperpigmentation and facial pigmentation arise due to vitiation of Pitta, Rakta, and Bhrajaka Pitta affecting skin complexion. Ayurveda offers holistic management through blood purification, herbal therapies, Panchakarma, proper skincare, and dietary regulation. Timely Ayurvedic treatment helps restore natural complexion, reduce discoloration, and improve overall skin health naturally.

Chapter 7

MELASMA & POST-INFLAMMATORY HYPERPIGMENTATION

Introduction

Melasma and post-inflammatory hyperpigmentation are chronic pigmentation disorders characterized by brown, gray, or dark patches over the face following hormonal changes, sun exposure, acne, inflammation, or skin injury. In Ayurveda, these conditions are primarily associated with vitiation of Pitta, Rakta, and Bhrajaka Pitta affecting skin complexion and pigmentation balance.

Classical Reference (श्लोक)

"पित्तदूषितरक्तेन त्वचो वर्णविपर्ययः ।
श्याववर्णा भवेत् त्वचा दाहयुक्ता विशेषतः ॥"

— Ayurvedic Classical Reference

Meaning

Vitiated Pitta and Rakta produce abnormal dark discoloration of the skin often associated with burning sensation.

Another reference:

"भ्राजकपित्तवैषम्यात् मुखवर्णविकृतिः भवेत्।"

Meaning: Disturbance of Bhrajaka Pitta causes abnormal facial complexion and pigmentation.

Nidana (Causes)

- Excess sun exposure
- Hormonal imbalance
- Pregnancy and oral contraceptives
- Acne and inflammatory skin disorders
- Excess cosmetic use
- Stress and emotional disturbances
- Excess spicy and sour food
- Sleep deprivation
- Nutritional deficiencies
- Chronic digestive disorders

Samprapti (Pathogenesis)

Aggravated Pitta vitiates Rakta and Bhrajaka Pitta in the skin, leading to excessive melanin deposition. Inflammatory skin conditions further damage skin tissues causing post-inflammatory pigmentation. Vata contributes to unevenness and dryness while Kapha causes dullness.

Lakshana (Symptoms)

- Brown or gray facial patches
- Pigmentation over cheeks, forehead, nose
- Dark marks after acne or inflammation
- Uneven complexion
- Dull skin
- Mild burning sensation
- Recurrence after sun exposure

Ayurvedic Management

1. Shamana Chikitsa (Internal Medicines)

Mahamanjishthadi Kwath

Dosage: 15–20 ml twice daily
Anupana: Equal quantity of water
Duration: 3 months

Khadirarishta

Dosage: 15–20 ml twice daily after meals
Anupana: Equal quantity of water
Duration: 2–3 months

Sarivadyasava

Dosage: 15–20 ml twice daily
Anupana: Equal quantity of water
Duration: 2 months

Gandhak Rasayan

Dosage: 250 mg twice daily
Anupana: Honey
Duration: 2 months

Avipattikar Churna

Dosage: 3–5 grams at bedtime
Anupana: Warm water
Duration: 1–2 months

2. External Therapies

Mukhalepa (Face Pack)

Ingredients:

- Manjistha
- Yashtimadhu

- Sandalwood
- Lodhra
- Turmeric

Apply daily or alternate days for 20–30 minutes.

Kumkumadi Taila

Night application helps improve complexion and reduce pigmentation.

Aloe Vera Gel

Useful in soothing inflamed and pigmented skin.

3. Panchakarma

Virechana

Most beneficial for Pitta-dominant pigmentation disorders.

Raktamokshana

Useful in chronic and recurrent pigmentation.

Nasya

Improves facial nourishment and complexion.

Pathya (Wholesome Diet & Lifestyle)

Recommended Foods

- Amla
- Coconut water
- Pomegranate
- Green vegetables

- Bitter vegetables
- Mung dal
- Cow's ghee
- Fresh fruits

Healthy Practices

- Daily sun protection
- Adequate hydration
- Stress reduction
- Proper sleep
- Gentle skincare
- Yoga and meditation

Apathya (To Avoid)

- Excess sunlight exposure
- Spicy, sour, fried foods
- Harsh chemical cosmetics
- Excess tea and coffee
- Smoking and alcohol
- Late-night sleeping
- Excess stress and anger

Prognosis (Sadhya-Asadhyata)

- Mild and recent pigmentation: Sadhya (curable)
- Chronic melasma: Yapya (manageable)
- Regular treatment and sun protection improve outcomes significantly.

Conclusion

Melasma and post-inflammatory hyperpigmentation result from vitiation of Pitta, Rakta, and Bhrajaka Pitta causing abnormal pigmentation and discoloration. Ayurveda provides holistic management through blood purification, herbal medicines, Panchakarma, dietary correction, and skin rejuvenation therapies. Timely Ayurvedic care helps reduce pigmentation, improve complexion, and maintain healthy radiant skin naturally.

Chapter 8

DARK CIRCLES, FACIAL DULLNESS & LOSS OF GLOW

Introduction

Dark circles, facial dullness, and loss of natural glow are common cosmetic concerns resulting from stress, lack of sleep, nutritional deficiency, excessive screen exposure, and improper lifestyle. In Ayurveda, these conditions are associated with imbalance of Vata, Pitta, Rakta, and Rasa Dhatu. Poor circulation, tissue depletion, and aggravated Pitta around the eyes and facial skin lead to discoloration and reduced radiance.

Classical Reference (श्लोक)

"रक्तक्षये त्वचो वर्णः श्यावता याति देहिनाम् ।
वातपित्तप्रकोपाच्च कान्तिहानिर्भवेद्ध्रुवम् ॥"

— Ayurvedic Classical Reference

Meaning

Depletion of Rakta along with aggravation of Vata and Pitta causes dark discoloration and loss of complexion.

Another reference:

"रसधातुक्षये कान्तिर्हीयते शरीरिणाम् ।"

Meaning: Depletion of Rasa Dhatu leads to loss of glow and vitality.

Nidana (Causes)

- Sleep deprivation
- Stress and anxiety
- Excess screen exposure
- Nutritional deficiency
- Chronic illness and weakness
- Excessive mental work
- Dehydration
- Irregular food habits
- Excess sun exposure
- Smoking and alcohol

Samprapti (Pathogenesis)

Aggravated Vata causes dryness and poor circulation around the eyes and facial skin. Pitta vitiates Rakta leading to dark discoloration, while depletion of Rasa Dhatu reduces skin nourishment and glow. Chronic stress further aggravates tissue depletion.

Lakshana (Symptoms)

- Dark circles under eyes
- Facial dullness
- Tired appearance
- Dry and lifeless skin
- Uneven complexion
- Fine lines around eyes
- Reduced skin radiance

Ayurvedic Management

1. Shamana Chikitsa (Internal Medicines)

Amalaki Rasayana

Dosage: 3–5 grams twice daily
Anupana: Milk
Duration: 3 months

Saptamrit Lauha

Dosage: 250 mg twice daily
Anupana: Honey and ghee
Duration: 2–3 months

Brahmi Vati

(Useful in stress-related dullness)

Dosage: 1 tablet twice daily
Anupana: Water or milk
Duration: 2 months

Ashwagandha Churna

Dosage: 3–5 grams twice daily
Anupana: Milk
Duration: 2–3 months

2. External Therapies

Eye & Facial Applications

Kumkumadi Taila

Gentle nightly massage improves complexion and skin glow.

Cucumber & Aloe Vera Application

Useful for cooling and soothing dark circles.

Rose Water Compress

Helps refresh tired eyes and sensitive skin.

Chandan-Yashtimadhu Lepa

Improves complexion and reduces facial dullness.

3. Panchakarma

Nasya

Useful in improving facial circulation and nourishment.

Shirodhara

Beneficial in stress-related facial dullness and insomnia.

Abhyanga

Improves circulation and nourishes skin tissues.

Pathya (Wholesome Diet & Lifestyle)

Recommended Foods

- Amla
- Cow's ghee
- Almonds
- Walnuts
- Milk
- Fresh fruits
- Green vegetables
- Coconut water
- Mung dal

Healthy Practices

- Adequate sleep
- Stress management

- Yoga and meditation
- Eye relaxation exercises
- Proper hydration
- Regular facial massage

Apathya (To Avoid)

- Late-night sleeping
- Excess screen time
- Smoking and alcohol
- Excess tea and coffee
- Stress and anxiety
- Dehydration
- Junk and processed foods

Prognosis (Sadhya-Asadhyata)

- Mild dark circles and dullness: Sadhya (curable)
- Chronic hereditary dark circles: Yapya (manageable)
- Proper lifestyle correction gives excellent improvement.

Conclusion

Dark circles, facial dullness, and loss of glow reflect internal imbalance of Vata, Pitta, Rakta, and Rasa Dhatu along with lifestyle disturbances. Ayurveda offers holistic management through Rasayana therapy, stress reduction, Panchakarma, proper nutrition, and rejuvenating skin therapies. Timely Ayurvedic care helps restore natural radiance, freshness, and healthy glowing skin naturally.

Chapter 9

FACIAL REDNESS, ROSACEA & FLUSHING DISORDERS

Introduction

Facial redness, rosacea, and flushing disorders are chronic inflammatory skin conditions characterized by persistent redness, visible blood vessels, burning sensation, sensitivity, and episodic flushing of the face. In Ayurveda, these conditions are mainly associated with aggravation of Pitta and Rakta along with involvement of Bhrajaka Pitta in the skin. Heat, stress, spicy food, alcohol, and sun exposure commonly aggravate these disorders.

Classical Reference (श्लोक)

"पित्तेन रक्तदुष्टेन त्वचि दाहारुणं भवेत् ।
कण्डूशोफसमायुक्तं त्वग्विकारं प्रचक्षते ॥"

— Ayurvedic Classical Reference

Meaning

Vitiated Pitta and Rakta produce redness, burning, swelling, and inflammatory skin disorders.

Another reference:

"भ्राजकपित्तदोषेण मुखे रक्तिमा भवेत्।"

Meaning: Disturbance of Bhrajaka Pitta causes redness and discoloration on the face.

Nidana (Causes)

- Excess spicy and hot food
- Sun exposure and heat
- Emotional stress and anger
- Alcohol and smoking
- Excess tea and coffee
- Hormonal imbalance
- Harsh cosmetics
- Chronic digestive disturbances
- Hot climate exposure

Samprapti (Pathogenesis)

Aggravated Pitta vitiates Rakta and Bhrajaka Pitta in facial skin causing dilation of superficial blood vessels, redness, inflammation, and burning sensation. Vata contributes to hypersensitivity and dryness while Kapha may produce swelling and pustules.

Lakshana (Symptoms)

- Persistent facial redness
- Flushing episodes
- Burning sensation
- Facial warmth
- Visible tiny blood vessels
- Sensitive skin
- Acne-like eruptions

- Dryness and irritation

Ayurvedic Management

1. Shamana Chikitsa (Internal Medicines)

Mahatikta Ghrita

Dosage: 5–10 grams daily
Anupana: Warm water or milk
Duration: 2–3 months

Sarivadyasava

Dosage: 15–20 ml twice daily
Anupana: Equal quantity of water
Duration: 2 months

Mahamanjishthadi Kwath

Dosage: 15–20 ml twice daily
Anupana: Equal quantity of water
Duration: 3 months

Praval Pishti

Dosage: 125–250 mg twice daily
Anupana: Honey or ghee
Duration: 1–2 months

Avipattikar Churna

Dosage: 3–5 grams at bedtime
Anupana: Warm water
Duration: 1–2 months

2. External Therapies

Cooling Mukhalepa

Ingredients:

- Sandalwood
- Yashtimadhu
- Lodhra
- Rose petals
- Aloe vera

Apply daily for 20 minutes.

Rose Water Compress

Useful in reducing burning and redness.

Kumkumadi Taila

Gentle application improves skin texture and complexion.

3. Panchakarma

Virechana

Best therapy for Pitta-Rakta dominant rosacea.

Raktamokshana

Highly beneficial in chronic redness and inflammatory flushing disorders.

Shirodhara

Useful in stress-induced flushing and facial sensitivity.

Pathya (Wholesome Diet & Lifestyle)

Recommended Foods

- Amla
- Coconut water
- Pomegranate
- Cow's ghee
- Cucumber
- Green vegetables
- Buttermilk
- Fresh fruits

Healthy Practices

- Avoid direct sun exposure
- Stress management
- Adequate hydration
- Yoga and meditation
- Gentle skincare
- Regular sleep

Apathya (To Avoid)

- Spicy, sour, and fried foods
- Alcohol and smoking
- Excess tea and coffee
- Hot and humid environments
- Harsh cosmetics
- Emotional stress and anger

- Excess sunlight exposure

Prognosis (Sadhya-Asadhyata)

- Mild facial redness and flushing: Sadhya (curable)
- Chronic rosacea: Yapya (manageable)
- Early treatment helps prevent progression and vascular damage.

Conclusion

Facial redness, rosacea, and flushing disorders primarily arise due to aggravation of Pitta, Rakta, and Bhrajaka Pitta causing chronic inflammation and vascular sensitivity. Ayurveda provides holistic treatment through cooling therapies, blood purification, Panchakarma, diet correction, and stress management. Proper Ayurvedic care helps reduce redness, calm inflammation, and restore healthy balanced skin naturally.

PART 2

CHRONIC INFLAMMATORY & AUTOIMMUNE SKIN DISORDERS

Chapter 10

Eczema (Vicharchika) & Atopic Dermatitis

Introduction

Eczema and atopic dermatitis are chronic inflammatory skin disorders characterized by itching, dryness, redness, scaling, and recurrent skin irritation. In Ayurveda, eczema is closely correlated with **Vicharchika**, a type of Kshudra Kushta caused by vitiation of Kapha, Pitta, and Rakta along with involvement of Twak, Rakta, and Lasika. Chronic itching and recurrent inflammation significantly affect quality of life.

Classical Reference (श्लोक)

"कण्डूपिडकाभिः श्यावैः स्राविणीभिः समन्विता ।
विचर्चिका कफपित्तरक्तदुष्टिसमुद्भवा ॥"

— Ayurvedic Classical Reference

Meaning

Vicharchika is characterized by itching, eruptions, discoloration, and discharge caused by vitiation of Kapha, Pitta, and Rakta.

Another reference:

"कफात् कण्डूः पित्ततो दाहः त्वचि विकारकारकौ।"

Meaning: Kapha causes itching while Pitta produces burning and inflammation in skin disorders.

Nidana (Causes)

- Allergic tendency
- Excess intake of incompatible foods
- Excess spicy and oily foods
- Stress and anxiety
- Dust and environmental allergens
- Chemical exposure
- Digestive disturbances
- Irregular lifestyle
- Family history of allergy
- Excess sweating

Samprapti (Pathogenesis)

Aggravated Kapha and Pitta vitiate Rakta and Twak Dhatu causing inflammation, itching, and discharge. Vata contributes to dryness, fissuring, and chronicity. Repeated exposure to allergens aggravates immune hypersensitivity and skin barrier dysfunction.

Lakshana (Symptoms)

- Intense itching
- Dry or oozing lesions
- Redness and inflammation
- Thickened skin
- Cracking and scaling
- Burning sensation
- Recurrent flare-ups
- Sleep disturbance due to itching

Ayurvedic Management

1. Shamana Chikitsa (Internal Medicines)

Arogyavardhini Vati

Dosage: 250–500 mg twice daily
Anupana: Lukewarm water
Duration: 2–3 months

Gandhak Rasayan

Dosage: 250–500 mg twice daily
Anupana: Honey
Duration: 3 months

Mahamanjishthadi Kwath

Dosage: 15–20 ml twice daily after meals
Anupana: Equal quantity of water
Duration: 3 months

Khadirarishta

Dosage: 15–20 ml twice daily
Anupana: Equal quantity of water
Duration: 2–3 months

Panchatikta Ghrita

Dosage: 5–10 grams daily
Anupana: Warm water or milk
Duration: 2 months

2. External Therapies

Herbal Applications

Neem & Turmeric Paste

Useful in itching and inflammation.

Jatyadi Taila

Helpful in dry, cracked, and chronic lesions.

Coconut Oil Application

Provides soothing and moisturization in dry eczema.

Triphala Wash

Useful in cleansing oozing lesions.

3. Panchakarma

Virechana

Best for Pitta-Rakta dominant eczema.

Raktamokshana

Useful in chronic inflammatory eczema.

Vamana

Beneficial in Kapha-dominant oozing eczema.

Pathya (Wholesome Diet & Lifestyle)

Recommended Foods

- Neem preparations
- Amla
- Green vegetables
- Bitter vegetables

- Mung dal
- Buttermilk
- Coconut water
- Warm water

Healthy Practices

- Regular moisturization
- Stress management
- Yoga and meditation
- Gentle herbal cleansers
- Proper sleep
- Avoid excessive scratching

Apathya (To Avoid)

- Spicy, oily, and sour foods
- Seafood and incompatible foods
- Excess sweets and dairy
- Harsh soaps and chemicals
- Smoking and alcohol
- Stress and anxiety
- Dust and allergens

Prognosis (Sadhya-Asadhyata)

- Mild and recent eczema: Sadhya (curable)
- Chronic recurrent eczema: Yapya (manageable)
- Early treatment helps prevent chronic thickening and secondary infection.

Conclusion

Eczema and atopic dermatitis arise due to vitiation of Kapha, Pitta, Rakta, and Vata causing chronic inflammation, itching, and skin barrier dysfunction. Ayurveda offers holistic management through purification therapies, blood purification, herbal medicines, dietary regulation, and lifestyle correction. Proper Ayurvedic care helps reduce recurrence, improve skin healing, and restore healthy skin naturally.

Chapter 11

CONTACT & SEBORRHEIC DERMATITIS

Introduction

Contact dermatitis and seborrheic dermatitis are inflammatory skin disorders characterized by redness, itching, scaling, irritation, and oily or dry flaky lesions. Contact dermatitis occurs due to exposure to allergens or irritants, while seborrheic dermatitis commonly affects oily areas such as scalp, face, and chest. In Ayurveda, these conditions are associated with vitiation of Kapha, Pitta, Rakta, and Vata affecting Twak and Lasika.

Classical Reference (श्लोक)

"कफपित्तप्रकोपेन त्वचि कण्डू रजः स्रवः ।
दाहशोफसमायुक्ता विकाराः सम्भवन्ति हि ॥"

— Ayurvedic Classical Reference

Meaning

Aggravation of Kapha and Pitta causes itching, scaling, discharge, inflammation, and swelling in skin disorders.

Another reference:

"दूषितं रक्तमाश्रित्य पित्तं त्वचि विकारकृत्।"

Meaning: Vitiated Pitta affecting Rakta produces inflammatory skin diseases.

Nidana (Causes)

Contact Dermatitis

- Chemical exposure
- Cosmetics and hair dyes
- Detergents and soaps
- Metal allergy
- Dust and environmental allergens

Seborrheic Dermatitis

- Excess oil secretion
- Stress and anxiety
- Poor scalp hygiene
- Humid climate
- Digestive disturbances
- Excess spicy and oily food

Samprapti (Pathogenesis)

Aggravated Pitta and Rakta produce inflammation and redness, while Kapha causes oiliness, itching, and scaling. Vata contributes to dryness and flaking. External allergens or excessive sebum disturb skin channels leading to chronic irritation and dermatitis.

Lakshana (Symptoms)

- Red inflamed patches
- Itching and irritation
- Oily or dry scales
- Flaky scalp and dandruff
- Burning sensation

- Crusting or discharge
- Skin sensitivity
- Recurrent flare-ups

Ayurvedic Management

1. Shamana Chikitsa (Internal Medicines)

Gandhak Rasayan

Dosage: 250–500 mg twice daily
Anupana: Honey
Duration: 2–3 months

Arogyavardhini Vati

Dosage: 250 mg twice daily
Anupana: Lukewarm water
Duration: 2 months

Khadirarishta

Dosage: 15–20 ml twice daily after meals
Anupana: Equal quantity of water
Duration: 2–3 months

Mahamanjishthadi Kwath

Dosage: 15–20 ml twice daily
Anupana: Equal quantity of water
Duration: 3 months

Panchatikta Ghrita

Dosage: 5–10 grams daily
Anupana: Warm water or milk
Duration: 2 months

2. External Therapies

For Contact Dermatitis

Sandalwood & Yashtimadhu Paste

Useful in redness and burning.

Coconut Oil Application

Helps soothe irritated skin.

For Seborrheic Dermatitis

Neem Taila / Nimbadi Taila

Useful in scalp scaling and itching.

Triphala or Neem Wash

Helps cleanse scalp and affected skin.

Aloe Vera Gel

Useful in soothing inflamed skin.

3. Panchakarma

Virechana

Best therapy for Pitta-dominant dermatitis.

Vamana

Useful in Kapha-dominant seborrheic dermatitis.

Raktamokshana

Beneficial in chronic inflammatory cases.

Pathya (Wholesome Diet & Lifestyle)

Recommended Foods

- Neem preparations
- Amla
- Green vegetables
- Bitter vegetables
- Buttermilk
- Coconut water
- Mung dal
- Warm water

Healthy Practices

- Maintain proper hygiene
- Use mild herbal cleansers
- Manage stress
- Keep scalp clean
- Adequate sleep
- Avoid known allergens

Apathya (To Avoid)

- Harsh soaps and cosmetics
- Hair dyes and chemical products
- Spicy and oily foods
- Excess sweets and dairy
- Smoking and alcohol
- Stress and sleep deprivation
- Excess sweating and humidity

Prognosis (Sadhya-Asadhyata)

- Mild dermatitis: Sadhya (curable)
- Chronic recurrent seborrheic dermatitis: Yapya (manageable)
- Avoidance of triggers improves long-term control.

Conclusion

Contact and seborrheic dermatitis arise due to vitiation of Kapha, Pitta, Rakta, and Vata causing chronic inflammation, itching, and scaling. Ayurveda offers holistic management through Dosha balancing, purification therapies, herbal medicines, skincare regulation, and lifestyle correction. Proper Ayurvedic treatment helps reduce recurrence, soothe irritation, and restore healthy skin naturally.

Chapter 12

PSORIASIS (KITIBHA KUSHTA)

Introduction

Psoriasis is a chronic autoimmune inflammatory skin disorder characterized by thick, dry, scaly plaques associated with itching and recurrent flare-ups. In Ayurveda, psoriasis is commonly correlated with **Kitibha Kushta**, a type of Kshudra Kushta caused by vitiation of Vata and Kapha along with involvement of Pitta and Rakta. Improper diet, stress, toxins, and immune dysregulation play important roles in its manifestation.

Classical Reference (श्लोक)

श्यावं किणखरस्पर्शं परुषं रूक्षमेव च।
किटिभं नाम कुष्ठं स्यात् वातकफसमुद्भवम्॥

— Charaka Samhita

Meaning

Kitibha Kushta is characterized by dark, rough, dry, hard, and scaly skin lesions caused predominantly by aggravated Vata and Kapha.

Another reference:

"कफवातप्रकोपेन त्वचि शुष्कत्वमुत्थितम्।"

Meaning: Aggravation of Kapha and Vata produces dryness, scaling, and thickening of skin.

Nidana (Causes)

- Incompatible food combinations
- Excess spicy, sour, and oily food
- Stress and anxiety
- Suppression of natural urges
- Alcohol and smoking
- Chronic digestive disturbances
- Genetic predisposition
- Irregular sleep
- Excess intake of curd and seafood together

Samprapti (Pathogenesis)

Aggravated Vata and Kapha vitiate Twak, Rakta, Mamsa, and Lasika leading to dryness, scaling, thickened plaques, and itching. Pitta contributes to redness and inflammation. Chronic toxin accumulation and immune dysfunction further aggravate recurrent lesions.

Lakshana (Symptoms)

- Thick scaly plaques
- Dry rough skin
- Silvery scales
- Itching
- Cracking and bleeding
- Red inflamed patches
- Burning sensation
- Recurrent flare-ups

Ayurvedic Management

1. Shamana Chikitsa (Internal Medicines)

Arogyavardhini Vati

Dosage: 250–500 mg twice daily
Anupana: Lukewarm water
Duration: 3 months

Panchatikta Ghrita Guggulu

Dosage: 1–2 tablets twice daily
Anupana: Warm water
Duration: 3–6 months

Mahamanjishthadi Kwath

Dosage: 15–20 ml twice daily after meals
Anupana: Equal quantity of water
Duration: 3 months

Khadirarishta

Dosage: 15–20 ml twice daily
Anupana: Equal quantity of water
Duration: 3 months

Gandhak Rasayan

Dosage: 250 mg twice daily
Anupana: Honey
Duration: 2–3 months

2. External Therapies

Herbal Applications

Mahamarichyadi Taila

Useful in thick scaly lesions.

Neem Oil Application

Helps reduce itching and inflammation.

Aloe Vera Gel

Provides soothing and moisturization.

Medicated Bath

Bathing with neem or Triphala decoction helps cleanse lesions.

3. Panchakarma

Virechana

Best for Pitta-Rakta involvement.

Vamana

Useful in Kapha-dominant psoriasis.

Raktamokshana

Beneficial in chronic inflammatory lesions.

Basti

Useful in chronic Vata-dominant dryness and scaling.

Pathya (Wholesome Diet & Lifestyle)

Recommended Foods

- Neem preparations

- Bitter vegetables
- Amla
- Green vegetables
- Mung dal
- Old barley and wheat
- Coconut water
- Warm water

Healthy Practices

- Regular oil massage
- Stress management
- Yoga and meditation
- Adequate sleep
- Gentle skin moisturization
- Daily exercise

Apathya (To Avoid)

- Curd and seafood combination
- Excess spicy and sour food
- Fermented foods
- Alcohol and smoking
- Stress and anxiety
- Junk food
- Excess sweets and dairy
- Late-night sleeping

Prognosis (Sadhya-Asadhyata)

- Mild psoriasis: Krichra Sadhya (difficult but curable)
- Chronic extensive psoriasis: Yapya (manageable)
- Long-term lifestyle and dietary discipline are essential.

Conclusion

Psoriasis (Kitibha Kushta) is a chronic autoimmune skin disorder caused by vitiation of Vata, Kapha, Pitta, and Rakta affecting deeper tissues. Ayurveda offers holistic management through purification therapies, blood purification, herbal medicines, Panchakarma, dietary correction, and lifestyle regulation. Proper Ayurvedic care helps control flare-ups, reduce scaling and itching, and improve quality of life naturally.

Chapter 13

VITILIGO (SHWITRA)

Introduction

Vitiligo is a chronic depigmentary skin disorder characterized by white patches due to loss of skin pigmentation. In Ayurveda, vitiligo is correlated with **Shwitra**, a type of Kushta caused by vitiation of Tridosha, predominantly Pitta, along with Rakta, Mamsa, and Meda Dushti. Improper diet, incompatible food combinations, stress, and autoimmune disturbances are important contributing factors.

Classical Reference (श्लोक)

"श्वित्रं तु त्रिदोषजं प्रोक्तं त्वग्मांसासृगाश्रयम् ।
वर्णभेदकरं रोगं कठिनं चिरसंस्थितम् ॥"

— Charaka Samhita

Meaning

Shwitra is a Tridoshaja disorder affecting skin, blood, and muscle tissues causing discoloration and chronic depigmented patches.

Another reference:

"विरुद्धाहारसेवनात् कुष्ठानि प्रजायन्ते।"

Meaning: Consumption of incompatible foods leads to skin disorders including Shwitra.

Nidana (Causes)

- Incompatible food combinations
- Excess sour and salty foods
- Fish with milk intake
- Autoimmune tendency
- Stress and emotional trauma
- Chronic digestive disturbances
- Genetic predisposition
- Excessive sun exposure
- Suppression of natural urges

Samprapti (Pathogenesis)

Aggravated Pitta along with Vata and Kapha vitiates Rakta, Mamsa, and Meda Dhatu leading to destruction of skin pigmentation. Impaired Bhrajaka Pitta causes depigmented white patches. Chronic immune dysfunction and toxin accumulation aggravate disease progression.

Lakshana (Symptoms)

- White depigmented patches
- Gradual spread of lesions
- Hair whitening over patches
- Mild itching occasionally
- Cosmetic disfigurement
- Irregular patch margins
- Sensitivity to sunlight

Ayurvedic Management

1. Shamana Chikitsa (Internal Medicines)

Bakuchi Churna

Dosage: 1–3 grams twice daily
Anupana: Honey or warm water
Duration: 3–6 months

Khadirarishta

Dosage: 15–20 ml twice daily after meals
Anupana: Equal quantity of water
Duration: 3 months

Mahamanjishthadi Kwath

Dosage: 15–20 ml twice daily
Anupana: Equal quantity of water
Duration: 3 months

Arogyavardhini Vati

Dosage: 250 mg twice daily
Anupana: Lukewarm water
Duration: 2–3 months

Gandhak Rasayan

Dosage: 250 mg twice daily
Anupana: Honey
Duration: 2 months

2. External Therapies

Bakuchi Taila Application

Applied carefully over depigmented patches under supervision.

Neem & Manjistha Paste

Useful in skin purification.

Controlled Sun Exposure

Mild early morning sunlight exposure helps pigmentation.

3. Panchakarma

Virechana

Best therapy for Pitta-dominant Shwitra.

Raktamokshana

Useful in chronic and spreading lesions.

Vamana

Indicated in Kapha-dominant cases.

Pathya (Wholesome Diet & Lifestyle)

Recommended Foods

- Neem preparations
- Amla
- Bitter vegetables
- Green leafy vegetables
- Old grains
- Mung dal
- Cow's ghee
- Warm water

Healthy Practices

- Stress management

- Yoga and meditation
- Regular digestion maintenance
- Proper sleep
- Gentle skincare
- Daily exercise

Apathya (To Avoid)

- Fish with milk
- Curd and sour foods
- Excess salty and spicy foods
- Fermented foods
- Alcohol and smoking
- Stress and anxiety
- Junk food
- Excess sunlight exposure

Prognosis (Sadhya-Asadhyata)

- Recent and localized Shwitra: Krichra Sadhya (difficult but curable)
- Chronic widespread vitiligo: Yapya (manageable)
- Early treatment improves chances of repigmentation.

Conclusion

Vitiligo (Shwitra) is a chronic depigmentary disorder caused by Tridosha imbalance affecting Rakta, Mamsa, and Bhrajaka Pitta. Ayurveda offers holistic management through purification therapies, herbal medicines, dietary discipline, Panchakarma, and lifestyle correction. Timely Ayurvedic intervention helps control disease progression, improve pigmentation, and support healthy skin naturally.

Chapter 14

URTICARIA (SHEETAPITTA) & ALLERGIC SKIN DISORDERS

Introduction

Urticaria and allergic skin disorders are characterized by sudden appearance of itchy wheals, redness, swelling, burning sensation, and recurrent allergic reactions. In Ayurveda, urticaria is correlated with **Sheetapitta**, a disorder caused by vitiation of Vata and Pitta along with Rakta Dushti. Exposure to allergens, incompatible foods, stress, and weakened digestion commonly trigger these conditions.

Classical Reference (श्लोक)

"शीतपित्तं तु विज्ञेयं वातपित्तप्रकोपजम् ।
कण्डूदाहसमायुक्तं त्वचि शोफं प्रदर्शयेत् ॥"

— Ayurvedic Classical Reference

Meaning

Sheetapitta is caused by aggravation of Vata and Pitta producing itching, burning, and swelling over the skin.

Another reference:

"दूषितं रक्तमाश्रित्य पित्तं त्वचि विकारकृत्।"

Meaning: Vitiated Pitta affecting Rakta causes inflammatory and allergic skin manifestations.

Nidana (Causes)

- Food allergies
- Incompatible food combinations
- Dust, pollen, and environmental allergens
- Excess spicy and sour food
- Stress and anxiety
- Drug reactions
- Cold exposure or sudden temperature changes
- Digestive disturbances
- Insect bites

Samprapti (Pathogenesis)

Aggravated Pitta and Vata vitiate Rakta and Twak causing hypersensitivity reactions in skin. Kapha may contribute to swelling and heaviness. Impaired digestion and toxin accumulation increase allergic tendencies and recurrent flare-ups.

Lakshana (Symptoms)

- Raised itchy wheals
- Redness and swelling
- Burning sensation
- Sudden allergic eruptions
- Skin irritation
- Recurrent episodes
- Pruritus
- Heat or cold sensitivity

Ayurvedic Management

1. Shamana Chikitsa (Internal Medicines)

Haridra Khanda

Dosage: 3–5 grams twice daily
Anupana: Milk or warm water
Duration: 2–3 months

Gandhak Rasayan

Dosage: 250–500 mg twice daily
Anupana: Honey
Duration: 2 months

Mahamanjishthadi Kwath

Dosage: 15–20 ml twice daily
Anupana: Equal quantity of water
Duration: 2–3 months

Avipattikar Churna

Dosage: 3–5 grams at bedtime
Anupana: Warm water
Duration: 1–2 months

Kamdudha Ras

Dosage: 125–250 mg twice daily
Anupana: Ghee or honey
Duration: 1–2 months

2. External Therapies

Cooling Applications

Sandalwood Paste

Useful in burning and redness.

Neem & Turmeric Paste

Helps reduce itching and allergic inflammation.

Rose Water Compress

Provides cooling and soothing effect.

Coconut Oil Application

Useful in dry allergic skin conditions.

3. Panchakarma

Virechana

Best therapy for Pitta-dominant allergic disorders.

Raktamokshana

Useful in chronic recurrent urticaria.

Vamana

Indicated in Kapha-associated allergic conditions.

Pathya (Wholesome Diet & Lifestyle)

Recommended Foods

- Amla
- Neem preparations
- Coconut water
- Pomegranate
- Green vegetables
- Mung dal
- Cow's ghee
- Warm water

Healthy Practices

- Avoid known allergens
- Maintain digestive health
- Adequate hydration
- Stress management
- Yoga and meditation
- Regular sleep

Apathya (To Avoid)

- Seafood and incompatible foods
- Spicy, sour, and fried foods
- Fermented foods
- Excess tea and coffee
- Smoking and alcohol
- Stress and anxiety
- Cold drinks and ice cream

Prognosis (Sadhya-Asadhyata)

- Acute urticaria: Sadhya (curable)
- Chronic recurrent allergic disorders: Yapya (manageable)
- Trigger avoidance improves long-term outcomes.

Conclusion

Urticaria (Sheetapitta) and allergic skin disorders arise due to vitiation of Vata, Pitta, Rakta, and impaired immunity causing hypersensitivity reactions in skin. Ayurveda provides holistic management through purification therapies, blood purification, anti-allergic herbs, dietary regulation, and lifestyle correction. Proper Ayurvedic care helps reduce recurrence, calm allergic reactions, and maintain healthy skin naturally.

Chapter 15

CHRONIC PRURITUS & XEROTIC SKIN DISORDERS

Introduction

Chronic pruritus (persistent itching) and xerotic skin disorders (abnormally dry skin conditions) are common dermatological problems associated with dryness, roughness, scaling, irritation, and recurrent itching. In Ayurveda, these conditions are mainly caused by aggravation of Vata Dosha along with involvement of Pitta and Rakta. Deficiency of skin lubrication, aging, excessive washing, nutritional deficiency, and environmental dryness commonly contribute to these disorders.

Classical Reference (श्लोक)

"वातप्रकोपात् त्वक् रूक्षा खरस्पर्शा च जायते ।
कण्डूयुक्ता विवर्णा च त्वग्विकाराः प्रजायते ॥"

— Ayurvedic Classical Reference

Meaning

Aggravated Vata causes dry, rough, discolored skin associated with itching and skin disorders.

Another reference:

"रूक्षता वातलक्षणं त्वचि भेदकरं स्मृतम्।"

Meaning: Dryness caused by Vata leads to cracking and degeneration of the skin.

Nidana (Causes)

- Excessive dryness and cold climate
- Aging
- Nutritional deficiency
- Excessive bathing and harsh soaps
- Chronic stress and anxiety
- Sleep deprivation
- Dehydration
- Excess fasting
- Chronic illness
- Excess intake of dry and light foods

Samprapti (Pathogenesis)

Aggravated Vata dries the skin and depletes natural lubrication causing roughness, scaling, and fissuring. Pitta may produce burning and irritation, while Rakta Dushti contributes to itching and discoloration. Impaired nourishment of Rasa and Rakta Dhatu weakens skin integrity.

Lakshana (Symptoms)

- Persistent itching
- Dry rough skin
- Scaling and flaking
- Skin tightness
- Cracks and fissures
- Mild redness
- Burning sensation
- Sleep disturbance due to itching

Ayurvedic Management

1. Shamana Chikitsa (Internal Medicines)

Mahatikta Ghrita

Dosage: 5–10 grams daily
Anupana: Warm milk or water
Duration: 2–3 months

Gandhak Rasayan

Dosage: 250 mg twice daily
Anupana: Honey
Duration: 2 months

Manibhadra Guda

Dosage: 5–10 grams at bedtime
Anupana: Warm water
Duration: 1–2 months

Sarivadyasava

Dosage: 15–20 ml twice daily
Anupana: Equal quantity of water
Duration: 2 months

Ashwagandha Churna

Dosage: 3–5 grams twice daily
Anupana: Milk
Duration: 2–3 months

2. External Therapies

Oil Applications

Coconut Oil / Sesame Oil Massage

Useful in dryness and itching.

Mahamarichyadi Taila

Helpful in chronic dry skin lesions.

Aloe Vera Gel

Provides soothing hydration.

Oatmeal & Sandalwood Paste

Useful in calming irritated skin.

3. Panchakarma

Abhyanga

Daily oil massage is highly beneficial in Vata-dominant dry skin disorders.

Basti

Best therapy for chronic Vata aggravation.

Shirodhara

Useful in stress-related itching disorders.

Pathya (Wholesome Diet & Lifestyle)

Recommended Foods

- Cow's ghee
- Milk

- Almonds and walnuts
- Amla
- Fresh fruits
- Green vegetables
- Mung dal
- Coconut water

Healthy Practices

- Regular oil massage
- Adequate hydration
- Proper sleep
- Stress management
- Gentle herbal cleansers
- Yoga and meditation

Apathya (To Avoid)

- Excess dry and spicy foods
- Harsh soaps and hot water
- Excess fasting
- Smoking and alcohol
- Stress and anxiety
- Cold dry environments
- Late-night sleeping

Prognosis (Sadhya-Asadhyata)

- Mild xerotic skin disorders: Sadhya (curable)
- Chronic pruritus with systemic disease: Yapya (manageable)
- Regular moisturization and Vata balancing improve outcomes.

Conclusion

Chronic pruritus and xerotic skin disorders arise mainly due to Vata aggravation causing dryness, itching, and impaired skin nourishment. Ayurveda offers holistic management through oleation therapies, Rasayana treatment, Panchakarma, proper nutrition, and lifestyle correction. Timely Ayurvedic care helps restore skin hydration, reduce itching, and maintain healthy supple skin naturally.

Chapter 16

AUTOIMMUNE & IMMUNE DYSREGULATION SKIN DISORDERS

Introduction

Autoimmune and immune dysregulation skin disorders include chronic inflammatory conditions where the immune system mistakenly attacks healthy skin tissues leading to recurrent inflammation, discoloration, scaling, itching, and tissue damage. Conditions such as psoriasis, vitiligo, lupus-related dermatoses, and chronic allergic disorders fall under this category. In Ayurveda, these disorders are primarily related to Tridosha imbalance with predominance of Pitta, Rakta Dushti, Ama accumulation, and impaired immunity (Ojas Kshaya).

Classical Reference (श्लोक)

"दोषधातुमलानां च विकृतिः कुष्ठकारिणी ।
रक्तं त्वचं च दूष्यन्ति दीर्घकालप्रवर्तिनः ॥"

— Ayurvedic Classical Reference

Meaning

Vitiated Doshas, Dhatus, and metabolic toxins produce chronic skin disorders affecting blood and skin tissues.

Another reference:

"आमदोषसमायुक्ता व्याधयः कठिनाः स्मृताः ।"

Meaning: Disorders associated with Ama (toxins) become chronic and difficult to cure.

Nidana (Causes)

- Autoimmune tendency
- Chronic stress and anxiety
- Improper diet and incompatible foods
- Digestive impairment and Ama formation
- Genetic predisposition
- Sleep deprivation
- Environmental toxins
- Smoking and alcohol
- Recurrent infections
- Emotional disturbances

Samprapti (Pathogenesis)

Aggravated Doshas along with Ama vitiate Rakta, Twak, Mamsa, and immune functions. Pitta and Rakta produce inflammation and tissue destruction, Vata causes degeneration and chronicity, while Kapha contributes to thickening and obstruction. Ojas depletion weakens immune regulation resulting in recurrent autoimmune skin manifestations.

Lakshana (Symptoms)

- Chronic recurrent skin lesions
- Redness and inflammation
- Scaling or depigmentation
- Itching and burning
- Skin sensitivity
- Fatigue and weakness
- Slow healing
- Stress aggravation

Ayurvedic Management

1. Shamana Chikitsa (Internal Medicines)

Guduchi Satva

Dosage: 500 mg twice daily
Anupana: Honey or warm water
Duration: 3–6 months

Mahamanjishthadi Kwath

Dosage: 15–20 ml twice daily
Anupana: Equal quantity of water
Duration: 3 months

Panchatikta Ghrita Guggulu

Dosage: 1–2 tablets twice daily
Anupana: Warm water
Duration: 3–6 months

Gandhak Rasayan

Dosage: 250 mg twice daily
Anupana: Honey
Duration: 2–3 months

Ashwagandha Churna

Dosage: 3–5 grams twice daily
Anupana: Milk
Duration: 3 months

2. External Therapies

Herbal Applications

Neem & Manjistha Paste

Useful in chronic inflammatory lesions.

Mahatikta Ghrita Application

Helpful in dry autoimmune skin lesions.

Coconut Oil & Aloe Vera

Provide soothing and nourishment.

3. Panchakarma

Virechana

Best for Pitta-Rakta dominant autoimmune skin disorders.

Raktamokshana

Useful in chronic inflammatory conditions.

Basti

Beneficial in chronic Vata-dominant autoimmune disorders.

Rasayana Therapy

Improves immunity and tissue regeneration.

Pathya (Wholesome Diet & Lifestyle)

Recommended Foods

- Guduchi
- Amla
- Neem preparations
- Green vegetables
- Mung dal
- Cow's ghee

- Fresh fruits
- Warm water

Healthy Practices

- Stress management
- Yoga and meditation
- Adequate sleep
- Regular detoxification
- Gentle skincare
- Daily exercise

Apathya (To Avoid)

- Incompatible foods
- Spicy, sour, and fried foods
- Excess sweets and junk food
- Smoking and alcohol
- Stress and anger
- Sleep deprivation
- Sedentary lifestyle

Prognosis (Sadhya-Asadhyata)

- Mild autoimmune skin disorders: Krichra Sadhya (difficult but curable)
- Chronic severe autoimmune conditions: Yapya (manageable)
- Long-term treatment and lifestyle discipline are essential.

Conclusion

Autoimmune and immune dysregulation skin disorders result from Tridosha imbalance, Ama accumulation, Rakta Dushti, and impaired immunity. Ayurveda provides holistic management through detoxification, immune modulation, Rasayana therapy, Panchakarma, dietary correction, and stress management. Proper Ayurvedic care helps reduce flare-ups, improve immunity, and maintain healthier skin naturally.

Chapter 17

REACTIVE SENSITIVE SKIN & CHRONIC FACIAL INFLAMMATION

Introduction

Reactive sensitive skin and chronic facial inflammation are characterized by redness, burning, irritation, dryness, hypersensitivity, and intolerance to cosmetics or environmental triggers. These conditions commonly worsen with stress, pollution, excessive skincare products, and heat exposure. In Ayurveda, such disorders are mainly caused by aggravation of Pitta and Vata along with Rakta Dushti affecting Bhrajaka Pitta of the skin.

Classical Reference (श्लोक)

"पित्तदुष्टे त्वचि दाहो रक्तिमा स्पर्शनासहः ।
वातसंयोगतः शोषः संवेदनाधिकत्वकम् ॥"

— Ayurvedic Classical Reference

Meaning

Vitiated Pitta causes burning, redness, and intolerance of skin, while associated Vata produces dryness and hypersensitivity.

Another reference:

"भ्राजकपित्तवैषम्यात् त्वचो विकाराः प्रजायन्ते।"

Meaning: Disturbance of Bhrajaka Pitta leads to various skin disorders and facial sensitivity.

Nidana (Causes)

- Excess cosmetic procedures
- Chemical-based skincare products
- Pollution and environmental toxins
- Excess sun exposure
- Stress and anxiety
- Excess spicy and hot food
- Sleep deprivation
- Hormonal imbalance
- Over-exfoliation of skin

Samprapti (Pathogenesis)

Aggravated Pitta vitiates Rakta and Bhrajaka Pitta causing inflammation, redness, and burning sensation. Vata causes dryness, impaired skin barrier, and hypersensitivity. Continuous irritation weakens skin resilience leading to chronic facial inflammation.

Lakshana (Symptoms)

- Facial redness
- Burning sensation
- Dryness and irritation
- Tightness of skin
- Sensitivity to cosmetics
- Itching and stinging
- Flushing episodes
- Dull and inflamed skin

Ayurvedic Management

1. Shamana Chikitsa (Internal Medicines)

Mahatikta Ghrita

Dosage: 5–10 grams daily
Anupana: Warm milk or water
Duration: 2–3 months

Sarivadyasava

Dosage: 15–20 ml twice daily
Anupana: Equal quantity of water
Duration: 2 months

Praval Pishti

Dosage: 125–250 mg twice daily
Anupana: Honey or ghee
Duration: 1–2 months

Guduchi Satva

Dosage: 500 mg twice daily
Anupana: Honey or warm water
Duration: 2–3 months

Avipattikar Churna

Dosage: 3–5 grams at bedtime
Anupana: Warm water
Duration: 1–2 months

2. External Therapies

Cooling Facial Therapies

Sandalwood & Yashtimadhu Paste

Useful in burning and redness.

Aloe Vera Gel Application

Helps soothe inflamed sensitive skin.

Rose Water Compress

Provides cooling and hydration.

Kumkumadi Taila

Gentle night application improves skin nourishment.

3. Panchakarma

Virechana

Best therapy for Pitta-dominant facial inflammation.

Nasya

Improves facial nourishment and skin balance.

Shirodhara

Beneficial in stress-related facial sensitivity.

Pathya (Wholesome Diet & Lifestyle)

Recommended Foods

- Amla
- Coconut water
- Cow's ghee
- Cucumber
- Pomegranate
- Green vegetables

- Fresh fruits
- Mung dal

Healthy Practices

- Gentle skincare routine
- Stress management
- Adequate hydration
- Proper sleep
- Yoga and meditation
- Avoid excessive cosmetic use

Apathya (To Avoid)

- Harsh chemical cosmetics
- Excess spicy and sour foods
- Excess sun exposure
- Smoking and alcohol
- Hot water washing
- Emotional stress and anger
- Late-night sleeping

Prognosis (Sadhya-Asadhyata)

- Mild reactive sensitive skin: Sadhya (curable)
- Chronic inflammatory sensitive skin: Yapya (manageable)
- Early barrier repair improves long-term skin resilience.

Conclusion

Reactive sensitive skin and chronic facial inflammation arise mainly due to aggravation of Pitta, Vata, Rakta, and Bhrajaka Pitta causing hypersensitivity and chronic irritation. Ayurveda offers holistic management through cooling therapies, skin nourishment, Panchakarma, stress reduction, and lifestyle correction. Proper Ayurvedic care helps calm inflammation, restore skin barrier function, and maintain healthy balanced skin naturally.

Chapter 18

RECURRENT ECZEMA, PSORIASIS & ALLERGIC DERMATOSES

Introduction

Recurrent eczema, psoriasis, and allergic dermatoses are chronic relapsing inflammatory skin disorders marked by itching, redness, scaling, dryness, and periodic flare-ups. These conditions often persist for years and are aggravated by stress, allergens, improper diet, and immune dysfunction. In Ayurveda, such recurrent dermatoses are considered chronic forms of **Kushta Roga** involving Tridosha imbalance, especially Kapha, Pitta, Rakta Dushti, and Ama accumulation.

Classical Reference (श्लोक)

"कुष्ठानि सप्तधा प्रोक्ता दोषदूष्यसमुद्भवाः ।
दीर्घकालानुबन्धित्वात् कृच्छ्रसाध्यानि देहिनाम् ॥"

— Charaka Samhita

Meaning

Kushta disorders arise due to vitiation of Doshas and tissues and are chronic, difficult-to-manage skin diseases.

Another reference:

"आमदोषप्रकोपेन व्याधयः पुनरुद्भवाः ।"

Meaning: Aggravation of Ama leads to recurrent manifestation of diseases.

Nidana (Causes)

- Chronic allergic tendency
- Incompatible food combinations
- Stress and emotional disturbances
- Digestive impairment and Ama
- Environmental allergens
- Excess spicy and oily foods
- Sleep deprivation
- Smoking and alcohol
- Genetic predisposition
- Improper skin care

Samprapti (Pathogenesis)

Aggravated Doshas along with Ama vitiate Twak, Rakta, Lasika, and Mamsa causing chronic inflammation and recurrent lesions. Kapha produces itching and scaling, Pitta causes redness and burning, while Vata contributes to dryness, fissuring, and recurrence.

Lakshana (Symptoms)

- Recurrent itching
- Red inflamed patches
- Dryness and scaling
- Thickened skin
- Burning sensation
- Oozing lesions in some cases
- Seasonal flare-ups
- Stress-aggravated symptoms

Ayurvedic Management

1. Shamana Chikitsa (Internal Medicines)

Panchatikta Ghrita Guggulu

Dosage: 1–2 tablets twice daily
Anupana: Warm water
Duration: 3–6 months

Mahamanjishthadi Kwath

Dosage: 15–20 ml twice daily after meals
Anupana: Equal quantity of water
Duration: 3 months

Khadirarishta

Dosage: 15–20 ml twice daily
Anupana: Equal quantity of water
Duration: 3 months

Gandhak Rasayan

Dosage: 250–500 mg twice daily
Anupana: Honey
Duration: 2–3 months

Guduchi Satva

Dosage: 500 mg twice daily
Anupana: Honey or warm water
Duration: 3 months

2. External Therapies

Herbal Applications

Neem Oil Application

Useful in itching and recurrent inflammation.

Mahatikta Ghrita

Helpful in dry scaly lesions.

Jatyadi Taila

Useful in cracked and chronic lesions.

Triphala Wash

Helps cleanse affected skin.

3. Panchakarma

Virechana

Best for Pitta-Rakta dominant chronic dermatoses.

Vamana

Useful in Kapha-dominant recurrent skin disorders.

Raktamokshana

Beneficial in chronic inflammatory lesions.

Basti

Useful in chronic Vata-associated dryness and recurrence.

Pathya (Wholesome Diet & Lifestyle)

Recommended Foods

- Neem preparations
- Amla
- Bitter vegetables
- Green vegetables
- Mung dal

- Cow's ghee
- Coconut water
- Warm water

Healthy Practices

- Stress management
- Yoga and meditation
- Adequate sleep
- Daily exercise
- Proper digestion maintenance
- Gentle skincare

Apathya (To Avoid)

- Incompatible foods
- Spicy, oily, and sour foods
- Excess sweets and fermented foods
- Smoking and alcohol
- Stress and anxiety
- Harsh cosmetic products
- Late-night sleeping

Prognosis (Sadhya-Asadhyata)

- Mild recurrent dermatoses: Krichra Sadhya (difficult but curable)
- Chronic severe recurrent disorders: Yapya (manageable)
- Long-term discipline and trigger avoidance are essential.

Conclusion

Recurrent eczema, psoriasis, and allergic dermatoses result from chronic Dosha imbalance, Rakta Dushti, Ama accumulation, and immune dysregulation. Ayurveda offers holistic management through purification therapies, immune modulation, herbal medicines, Panchakarma, dietary regulation, and lifestyle correction. Proper Ayurvedic care helps reduce flare-ups, improve skin healing, and maintain long-term skin health naturally.

PART 3

INFECTIOUS SKIN DISORDERS

Chapter 19

FUNGAL SKIN INFECTIONS & DERMATOPHYTOSIS

Introduction

Fungal skin infections and dermatophytosis are contagious skin disorders caused by fungal invasion of the skin, scalp, nails, or body folds. Common manifestations include ringworm, itching, redness, scaling, and circular lesions. In Ayurveda, these disorders are correlated with **Dadru Kushta**, a Kapha-Pitta dominant skin disease involving Twak, Rakta, and Lasika Dushti.

Classical Reference (श्लोक)

कण्डू रक्तं सकिण्डं च मण्डलानि समुत्थितम् ।
दद्रुकुष्ठं विजानीयात् कफपित्तसमुद्भवम् ॥
— Charaka Samhita

Meaning

Dadru Kushta presents with itching, redness, circular lesions, and eruptions caused by aggravated Kapha and Pitta.

Another reference:

“कफात् कण्डूः पित्ततो रागः त्वचि मण्डलसम्भवः।”

Meaning: Kapha causes itching while Pitta produces redness and circular inflammatory lesions.

Nidana (Causes)

- Excess sweating
- Poor hygiene
- Humid climate
- Tight synthetic clothing
- Diabetes and low immunity

- Sharing contaminated clothes or towels
- Excess oily and sweet foods
- Obesity
- Excessive moisture retention

Samprapti (Pathogenesis)

Aggravated Kapha and Pitta vitiate Twak, Rakta, and Lasika causing itching, redness, scaling, and fungal proliferation. Moisture accumulation and impaired skin immunity promote chronic and recurrent fungal infections.

Lakshana (Symptoms)

- Circular red lesions
- Severe itching
- Scaling and flaking
- Burning sensation
- Oozing in some lesions
- Foul odor in body folds
- Recurrent infection
- Skin discoloration

Ayurvedic Management

1. Shamana Chikitsa (Internal Medicines)

Gandhak Rasayan

Dosage: 250–500 mg twice daily
Anupana: Honey
Duration: 2–3 months

Arogyavardhini Vati

Dosage: 250 mg twice daily
Anupana: Lukewarm water
Duration: 2 months

Khadirarishta

Dosage: 15–20 ml twice daily after meals
Anupana: Equal quantity of water
Duration: 2–3 months

Mahamanjishthadi Kwath

Dosage: 15–20 ml twice daily
Anupana: Equal quantity of water
Duration: 3 months

Nimbadi Churna

Dosage: 3 grams twice daily
Anupana: Warm water
Duration: 2 months

2. External Therapies

Herbal Applications

Nimbadi Taila

Useful in itching and fungal lesions.

Gandhak Ointment

Helps reduce fungal growth and scaling.

Neem & Turmeric Paste

Useful in inflammatory fungal lesions.

Triphala Wash

Helps cleanse affected skin.

3. Panchakarma

Virechana

Best for Pitta-Kapha dominant fungal disorders.

Vamana

Useful in chronic Kapha-dominant recurrent infections.

Raktamokshana

Beneficial in severe inflammatory lesions.

Pathya (Wholesome Diet & Lifestyle)

Recommended Foods

- Neem preparations
- Bitter vegetables
- Amla
- Green vegetables
- Mung dal
- Buttermilk
- Warm water
- Light digestible food

Healthy Practices

- Maintain skin dryness
- Wear loose cotton clothes
- Daily bathing and hygiene
- Regular exercise
- Proper blood sugar control
- Avoid sharing personal items

Apathya (To Avoid)

- Excess sweets and oily foods
- Curd and fermented foods
- Tight synthetic clothing
- Excess sweating and moisture
- Poor hygiene
- Smoking and alcohol
- Daytime sleeping

Prognosis (Sadhya-Asadhyata)

- Mild fungal infections: Sadhya (curable)
- Chronic recurrent dermatophytosis: Yapya (manageable)
- Hygiene and long-term care are essential to prevent recurrence.

Conclusion

Fungal skin infections and dermatophytosis (Dadru Kushta) arise due to Kapha-Pitta imbalance, moisture accumulation, and impaired skin immunity. Ayurveda offers holistic management through antifungal herbs, purification therapies, Panchakarma, dietary regulation, and hygiene correction. Proper Ayurvedic care helps control infection, reduce recurrence, and restore healthy skin naturally.

Chapter 20

TINEA PEDIS, INTERTRIGO & RECURRENT FUNGAL DISORDERS

Introduction

Tinea pedis (athlete's foot), intertrigo, and recurrent fungal infections commonly affect moist body areas such as feet, groin, underarms, and skin folds. These disorders present with itching, redness, scaling, foul odor, fissuring, and recurrent fungal growth. In Ayurveda, these conditions are considered forms of **Dadru Kushta** and Kapha-Pitta dominant skin disorders associated with excessive moisture, sweating, and impaired immunity.

Classical Reference (श्लोक)

कफपित्तसमुत्थानं कण्डूरागसमन्वितम् ।
मण्डलोत्थं त्वगुद्भूतं दद्रुकुष्ठं प्रचक्षते ॥
— Ayurvedic Classical Reference

Meaning

Dadru Kushta arises due to aggravated Kapha and Pitta causing itching, redness, and circular skin lesions.

Another reference:

"स्वेदाधिक्येन कफश्च त्वचि दोषान् प्रकोपयेत्।"

Meaning: Excess sweating aggravates Kapha and contributes to skin disorders.

Nidana (Causes)

- Excess sweating
- Obesity and skin folds
- Tight footwear and synthetic clothing
- Poor hygiene
- Diabetes mellitus
- Humid climate
- Excess oily and sweet foods
- Repeated moisture exposure
- Low immunity

Samprapti (Pathogenesis)

Aggravated Kapha and Pitta vitiate Twak and Rakta leading to excessive moisture, itching, redness, and fungal proliferation. Continuous dampness weakens skin integrity and promotes chronic recurrent infections.

Lakshana (Symptoms)

- Itching in skin folds or feet
- Red circular lesions
- Scaling and peeling skin
- Foul smell
- Cracks between toes
- Burning sensation
- Oozing lesions
- Recurrent fungal episodes

Ayurvedic Management

1. Shamana Chikitsa (Internal Medicines)

Gandhak Rasayan

Dosage: 250–500 mg twice daily
Anupana: Honey
Duration: 2–3 months

Khadirarishta

Dosage: 15–20 ml twice daily after meals
Anupana: Equal quantity of water
Duration: 2–3 months

Arogyavardhini Vati

Dosage: 250 mg twice daily
Anupana: Lukewarm water
Duration: 2 months

Nimbadi Churna

Dosage: 3 grams twice daily
Anupana: Warm water
Duration: 2 months

Mahamanjishthadi Kwath

Dosage: 15–20 ml twice daily
Anupana: Equal quantity of water
Duration: 3 months

2. External Therapies

Herbal Applications

Nimbadi Taila

Useful in itching and recurrent fungal lesions.

Neem & Turmeric Paste

Helps reduce inflammation and fungal growth.

Triphala Wash

Useful for cleansing affected areas.

Dusting with Herbal Powders

Keeps moist areas dry and prevents recurrence.

3. Panchakarma

Virechana

Best for Pitta-Kapha dominant recurrent fungal disorders.

Vamana

Useful in chronic Kapha-associated fungal infections.

Raktamokshana

Beneficial in severe inflammatory recurrent lesions.

Pathya (Wholesome Diet & Lifestyle)

Recommended Foods

- Bitter vegetables
- Neem preparations
- Amla
- Green vegetables
- Mung dal
- Buttermilk
- Warm water
- Light digestible food

Healthy Practices

- Keep skin folds dry

- Wear loose cotton clothes
- Change socks regularly
- Maintain proper hygiene
- Daily foot care
- Control blood sugar levels

Apathya (To Avoid)

- Excess sweets and bakery products
- Curd and fermented foods
- Tight synthetic clothing
- Damp footwear
- Poor hygiene
- Smoking and alcohol
- Excess daytime sleeping

Prognosis (Sadhya-Asadhyata)

- Mild fungal infections: Sadhya (curable)
- Chronic recurrent fungal disorders: Yapya (manageable)
- Proper hygiene and long-term preventive care are essential.

Conclusion

Tinea pedis, intertrigo, and recurrent fungal disorders arise due to Kapha-Pitta imbalance, excessive moisture, and impaired skin resistance. Ayurveda offers holistic management through antifungal herbs, purification therapies, Panchakarma, hygiene correction, and dietary regulation. Proper Ayurvedic care helps control infection, reduce recurrence, and maintain healthy skin naturally.

Chapter 21

BACTERIAL SKIN INFECTIONS, FURUNCULOSIS & CARBUNCLES

Introduction

Bacterial skin infections, furunculosis (boils), and carbuncles are inflammatory skin conditions characterized by painful pus-filled swellings caused by bacterial invasion of hair follicles and deeper skin tissues. In Ayurveda, these disorders are associated with **Pidaka**, **Vidradhi**, and Rakta-Pitta-Kapha Dushti involving inflammation, suppuration, and tissue damage. Poor hygiene, diabetes, low immunity, and excessive heat in the body commonly contribute to these conditions.

Classical Reference (श्लोक)

"दोषैर्दुष्टैः समुत्पन्नः शोफो दाहसमन्वितः ।
पक्वो विद्रधिरित्युक्तः पीडायुक्तो विशेषतः ॥"

— Sushruta Samhita

Meaning

Inflammatory swellings caused by vitiated Doshas associated with pain, burning, and suppuration are termed Vidradhi.

Another reference:

"पित्तरक्तप्रकोपेन पूयस्रावो प्रजायते।"

Meaning: Aggravation of Pitta and Rakta leads to pus formation and inflammatory skin lesions.

Nidana (Causes)

- Poor hygiene
- Excess sweating
- Diabetes mellitus
- Low immunity
- Excess spicy and oily foods
- Recurrent skin trauma
- Obesity
- Stress and fatigue
- Improper wound care

Samprapti (Pathogenesis)

Aggravated Pitta and Rakta produce inflammation and suppuration, while Kapha contributes to swelling and pus formation. Vata causes pain and spreading tendency. Impaired immunity and local tissue contamination result in recurrent bacterial infections.

Lakshana (Symptoms)

- Painful boils and swellings
- Red inflamed lesions
- Pus discharge
- Burning sensation
- Fever in severe infections
- Tenderness
- Multiple recurrent boils
- Foul-smelling discharge

Ayurvedic Management

1. Shamana Chikitsa (Internal Medicines)

Gandhak Rasayan

Dosage: 250–500 mg twice daily
Anupana: Honey
Duration: 2–3 months

Kaishore Guggulu

Dosage: 1–2 tablets twice daily
Anupana: Warm water
Duration: 2–3 months

Mahamanjishthadi Kwath

Dosage: 15–20 ml twice daily after meals
Anupana: Equal quantity of water
Duration: 3 months

Khadirarishta

Dosage: 15–20 ml twice daily
Anupana: Equal quantity of water
Duration: 2 months

Triphala Guggulu

Dosage: 1–2 tablets twice daily
Anupana: Warm water
Duration: 2 months

2. External Therapies

Herbal Applications

Jatyadi Taila

Useful in healing infected lesions.

Turmeric & Neem Paste

Helps reduce infection and inflammation.

Triphala Wash

Useful for cleansing wounds and boils.

Panchavalkala Decoction Wash

Promotes wound healing and purification.

3. Panchakarma

Virechana

Best for Pitta-Rakta dominant infections.

Raktamokshana

Useful in recurrent inflammatory boils and carbuncles.

Vamana

Beneficial in Kapha-dominant suppurative conditions.

Pathya (Wholesome Diet & Lifestyle)

Recommended Foods

- Neem preparations
- Amla
- Bitter vegetables
- Green vegetables
- Mung dal
- Coconut water
- Warm water
- Light digestible food

Healthy Practices

- Maintain proper hygiene

- Keep affected areas clean
- Daily bathing
- Proper diabetes control
- Stress management
- Adequate hydration

Apathya (To Avoid)

- Excess sweets and oily foods
- Spicy and fried foods
- Poor hygiene
- Smoking and alcohol
- Excess sweating
- Picking or squeezing boils
- Junk food

Prognosis (Sadhya-Asadhyata)

- Mild bacterial infections: Sadhya (curable)
- Recurrent furunculosis in diabetics: Yapya (manageable)
- Early treatment prevents deep tissue spread and complications.

Conclusion

Bacterial skin infections, furunculosis, and carbuncles arise due to vitiation of Pitta, Rakta, Kapha, and impaired immunity leading to inflammation and pus formation. Ayurveda provides holistic management through blood purification, antimicrobial herbs, wound healing therapies, Panchakarma, dietary regulation, and hygiene correction. Proper Ayurvedic care helps control infection, promote healing, and reduce recurrence naturally.

Chapter 22

FOLLICULITIS, ABSCESSES & RECURRENT BOILS

Introduction

Folliculitis, abscesses, and recurrent boils are inflammatory disorders involving infection of hair follicles and surrounding skin tissues. These conditions present with painful pustules, swelling, redness, pus formation, and recurrent skin eruptions. In Ayurveda, such disorders are associated with **Pidaka**, **Vidradhi**, and Rakta-Pitta-Kapha Dushti causing inflammation, suppuration, and obstruction of skin channels.

Classical Reference (श्लोक)

"पित्तरक्तकफैर्दुष्टैः शोफः पूयसमन्वितः ।
पीडायुक्तः स विज्ञेयः विद्रधिः परिकीर्तितः ॥"

— Ayurvedic Classical Reference

Meaning

Inflammatory swellings associated with vitiated Pitta, Rakta, and Kapha along with pus and pain are termed Vidradhi.

Another reference:

"कफात् पूयः पित्ततो दाहो वातात् पीडा प्रजायते।"

Meaning: Kapha causes pus formation, Pitta causes burning, and Vata produces pain.

Nidana (Causes)

- Poor hygiene

- Excess sweating
- Repeated shaving or friction
- Diabetes mellitus
- Low immunity
- Obesity
- Tight clothing
- Excess spicy and oily food
- Stress and fatigue

Samprapti (Pathogenesis)

Aggravated Pitta and Rakta produce inflammation and redness, Kapha causes pus accumulation and swelling, while Vata causes pain and recurrence. Blockage of hair follicles and impaired immunity promote repeated infections and abscess formation.

Lakshana (Symptoms)

- Painful pustules around hair follicles
- Red swollen boils
- Pus discharge
- Burning sensation
- Tenderness
- Recurrent abscess formation
- Fever in severe cases
- Localized warmth and swelling

Ayurvedic Management

1. Shamana Chikitsa (Internal Medicines)

Kaishore Guggulu

Dosage: 1–2 tablets twice daily
Anupana: Warm water
Duration: 2–3 months

Gandhak Rasayan

Dosage: 250–500 mg twice daily
Anupana: Honey
Duration: 2 months

Triphala Guggulu

Dosage: 1–2 tablets twice daily
Anupana: Warm water
Duration: 2 months

Mahamanjishthadi Kwath

Dosage: 15–20 ml twice daily after meals
Anupana: Equal quantity of water
Duration: 3 months

Khadirarishta

Dosage: 15–20 ml twice daily
Anupana: Equal quantity of water
Duration: 2 months

2. External Therapies

Herbal Applications

Jatyadi Taila

Useful in healing boils and abscesses.

Neem & Turmeric Paste

Helps reduce infection and inflammation.

Panchavalkala Wash

Useful for cleansing infected skin.

Warm Herbal Compress

Promotes drainage and healing of abscesses.

3. Panchakarma

Virechana

Best for Pitta-Rakta dominant suppurative skin disorders.

Raktamokshana

Useful in recurrent boils and inflammatory lesions.

Vamana

Beneficial in Kapha-dominant recurrent infections.

Pathya (Wholesome Diet & Lifestyle)

Recommended Foods

- Neem preparations
- Bitter vegetables
- Amla
- Green vegetables
- Mung dal
- Coconut water
- Warm water
- Light digestible food

Healthy Practices

- Maintain personal hygiene

- Wear loose cotton clothes
- Daily cleansing of affected areas
- Proper diabetes control
- Stress management
- Adequate hydration

Apathya (To Avoid)

- Excess sweets and oily foods
- Fried and spicy foods
- Tight synthetic clothing
- Poor hygiene
- Smoking and alcohol
- Repeated squeezing of boils
- Excess sweating

Prognosis (Sadhya-Asadhyata)

- Mild folliculitis and boils: Sadhya (curable)
- Chronic recurrent abscesses: Yapya (manageable)
- Early treatment helps prevent deep tissue infection and scarring.

Conclusion

Folliculitis, abscesses, and recurrent boils arise due to vitiation of Pitta, Rakta, Kapha, and impaired skin immunity causing suppuration and inflammation. Ayurveda offers holistic management through blood purification, antimicrobial herbs, Panchakarma, wound healing therapies, dietary regulation, and hygiene correction. Proper Ayurvedic care helps reduce recurrence, promote healing, and maintain healthy skin naturally.

Chapter 23

VIRAL SKIN DISORDERS

Introduction

Viral skin disorders include conditions such as herpes, warts, molluscum contagiosum, chickenpox-related eruptions, and viral exanthematous skin lesions. These disorders commonly present with vesicles, eruptions, itching, burning, pain, and recurrent outbreaks. In Ayurveda, viral skin disorders are understood under various categories of **Kushta**, **Visarpa**, and **Masaka**, involving vitiation of Pitta, Kapha, Rakta, and impaired immunity (Ojas Kshaya).

Classical Reference (श्लोक)

"पित्तरक्तप्रकोपेन विसर्पो दाहवान् भवेत् ।
शोफरागसमायुक्तः शीघ्रगामी विशेषतः ॥"

— Charaka Samhita

Meaning

Aggravated Pitta and Rakta produce rapidly spreading inflammatory skin eruptions associated with redness, swelling, and burning.

Another reference:

"ओजः क्षये शरीरस्य व्याधिक्षमता विनश्यति।"

Meaning: Loss of Ojas weakens the body's resistance to diseases.

Nidana (Causes)

- Viral exposure and infection
- Low immunity
- Stress and fatigue
- Improper diet and lifestyle
- Sleep deprivation
- Excess spicy and sour foods
- Poor hygiene
- Chronic illness
- Emotional stress

Samprapti (Pathogenesis)

Aggravated Pitta and Rakta produce inflammatory eruptions and burning sensation, while Kapha contributes to vesicle and wart formation. Ojas depletion weakens immunity, allowing recurrent viral manifestations and delayed healing.

Lakshana (Symptoms)

- Vesicular eruptions
- Warts or raised lesions
- Burning sensation
- Itching
- Pain or tenderness
- Fever in acute viral eruptions
- Recurrent outbreaks
- Skin discoloration after healing

Ayurvedic Management

1. Shamana Chikitsa (Internal Medicines)

Guduchi Satva

Dosage: 500 mg twice daily
Anupana: Honey or warm water
Duration: 2–3 months

Gandhak Rasayan

Dosage: 250–500 mg twice daily
Anupana: Honey
Duration: 2 months

Mahamanjishthadi Kwath

Dosage: 15–20 ml twice daily after meals
Anupana: Equal quantity of water
Duration: 2–3 months

Khadirarishta

Dosage: 15–20 ml twice daily
Anupana: Equal quantity of water
Duration: 2 months

Arogyavardhini Vati

Dosage: 250 mg twice daily
Anupana: Lukewarm water
Duration: 2 months

2. External Therapies

Herbal Applications

Neem Paste

Useful in viral eruptions and itching.

Aloe Vera Gel

Provides cooling and healing effect.

Jatyadi Taila

Useful in healing ulcerative lesions.

Turmeric Application

Helps reduce inflammation and secondary infection.

3. Panchakarma

Virechana

Best for Pitta-Rakta dominant viral skin disorders.

Raktamokshana

Useful in recurrent inflammatory lesions.

Rasayana Therapy

Improves immunity and tissue resistance.

Pathya (Wholesome Diet & Lifestyle)

Recommended Foods

- Guduchi
- Amla
- Neem preparations
- Coconut water
- Green vegetables
- Fresh fruits
- Mung dal
- Warm water

Healthy Practices

- Adequate rest
- Stress management
- Proper hygiene
- Yoga and meditation

- Adequate hydration
- Immune-strengthening lifestyle

Apathya (To Avoid)

- Spicy and fried foods
- Excess sour foods
- Smoking and alcohol
- Sleep deprivation
- Stress and anxiety
- Excessive sun exposure
- Junk food

Prognosis (Sadhya-Asadhyata)

- Mild viral skin disorders: Sadhya (curable)
- Recurrent viral infections due to low immunity: Yapya (manageable)
- Strong immunity improves long-term outcomes.

Conclusion

Viral skin disorders arise due to vitiation of Pitta, Rakta, Kapha, and weakened immunity leading to inflammatory and recurrent skin eruptions. Ayurveda offers holistic management through immune modulation, blood purification, antiviral herbs, Panchakarma, dietary correction, and lifestyle regulation. Proper Ayurvedic care helps reduce recurrence, improve healing, and maintain healthy skin naturally.

Chapter 24

NAIL DISORDERS & FUNGAL NAIL INFECTIONS

Introduction

Nail disorders and fungal nail infections are common conditions affecting the color, texture, thickness, and strength of nails. Fungal infections may cause brittle, thickened, discolored, and deformed nails, while nutritional deficiency and systemic diseases may also weaken nail health. In Ayurveda, nail disorders are associated with vitiation of Vata, Kapha, and Rakta along with impairment of Asthi Dhatu nourishment.

Classical Reference (श्लोक)

"नखा अस्थिमलाः प्रोक्ता दोषैर्दूष्यन्ति सर्वदा ।
वातात् शुष्का भवेन्नखाः कफात् स्थूलाः पित्तरागिणः ॥"

— Ayurvedic Classical Reference

Meaning

Nails are considered the waste product of Asthi Dhatu. Vata causes dryness and brittleness, Kapha causes thickening, while Pitta causes discoloration and inflammation.

Another reference:

"कफदोषप्रकोपेन नखेषु विकृतिः भवेत्।"

Meaning: Aggravated Kapha leads to deformity and thickening of nails.

Nidana (Causes)

- Fungal infection
- Poor hygiene
- Excess moisture exposure
- Diabetes mellitus
- Nutritional deficiency
- Tight footwear
- Low immunity
- Trauma to nails
- Excess chemical exposure

Samprapti (Pathogenesis)

Aggravated Kapha causes thickening and fungal growth in nails, while Pitta produces discoloration and inflammation. Vata leads to brittleness and cracking. Impaired Asthi Dhatu nourishment weakens nail structure and promotes chronic nail disorders.

Lakshana (Symptoms)

- Thickened nails
- Yellow or black discoloration
- Brittle and cracked nails
- Nail deformity
- Foul odor
- Pain or tenderness
- Separation of nail plate
- Rough nail surface

Ayurvedic Management

1. Shamana Chikitsa (Internal Medicines)

Gandhak Rasayan

Dosage: 250–500 mg twice daily
Anupana: Honey
Duration: 2–3 months

Kaishore Guggulu

Dosage: 1 tablet twice daily
Anupana: Warm water
Duration: 2–3 months

Arogyavardhini Vati

Dosage: 250 mg twice daily
Anupana: Lukewarm water
Duration: 2 months

Khadirarishta

Dosage: 15–20 ml twice daily after meals
Anupana: Equal quantity of water
Duration: 2 months

Lakshadi Guggulu

(Useful in weak and brittle nails)

Dosage: 1 tablet twice daily
Anupana: Warm milk
Duration: 3 months

2. External Therapies

Nail Applications

Nimbadi Taila

Useful in fungal nail infections.

Neem & Turmeric Paste

Helps reduce infection and discoloration.

Triphala Wash

Useful in cleansing infected nails.

Coconut Oil Application

Helps nourish brittle nails.

3. Panchakarma

Virechana

Best for Pitta-Kapha dominant nail disorders.

Raktamokshana

Useful in chronic inflammatory nail conditions.

Rasayana Therapy

Improves Asthi Dhatu nourishment and nail strength.

Pathya (Wholesome Diet & Lifestyle)

Recommended Foods

- Amla
- Sesame seeds

- Cow's ghee
- Milk
- Green vegetables
- Almonds
- Mung dal
- Warm water

Healthy Practices

- Maintain nail hygiene
- Keep nails dry
- Wear comfortable footwear
- Trim nails regularly
- Proper diabetes control
- Avoid nail trauma

Apathya (To Avoid)

- Excess moisture exposure
- Tight footwear
- Excess sweets and junk food
- Nail-biting habit
- Smoking and alcohol
- Harsh nail cosmetics
- Poor hygiene

Prognosis (Sadhya-Asadhyata)

- Mild fungal nail infections: Sadhya (curable)
- Chronic thickened nail disorders: Yapya (manageable)

- Long-term treatment and hygiene are essential.

Conclusion

Nail disorders and fungal nail infections arise due to vitiation of Vata, Kapha, Rakta, and impaired Asthi Dhatu nourishment. Ayurveda offers holistic management through antifungal herbs, Rasayana therapy, Panchakarma, nutritional support, and hygiene correction. Proper Ayurvedic care helps improve nail strength, reduce infection, and restore healthy nails naturally.

PART 4

COSMETIC, AGING & AESTHETIC DERMATOLOGY

Chapter 25

COSMETIC-INDUCED DERMATITIS & STEROID-DAMAGED SKIN

Introduction

Cosmetic-induced dermatitis and steroid-damaged skin are increasingly common skin disorders caused by prolonged use of chemical cosmetics, fairness creams, topical steroids, and harsh skincare products. These conditions present with redness, burning, thinning of skin, acne-like eruptions, pigmentation, and hypersensitivity. In Ayurveda, these disorders are associated with vitiation of Pitta, Rakta, and Bhrajaka Pitta along with weakening of skin tissues.

Classical Reference (श्लोक)

"पित्तदूषितरक्तेन त्वचि दाहो विवर्णता ।
शोफकण्डूसमन्विता त्वग्दुष्टिः सम्प्रजायते ॥"

— Ayurvedic Classical Reference

Meaning

Vitiated Pitta and Rakta produce burning, discoloration, swelling, itching, and damage to the skin.

Another reference:

"अतियोगात् भेषजानां विकाराः सम्भवन्ति हि।"

Meaning: Excessive or improper use of medicines can itself produce disorders.

Nidana (Causes)

- Excessive use of topical steroids
- Chemical cosmetics and fairness creams
- Frequent cosmetic procedures
- Harsh exfoliation
- Excess sun exposure
- Improper skincare routines
- Sensitive skin tendency
- Pollution and environmental toxins

Samprapti (Pathogenesis)

Aggravated Pitta and Rakta damage Bhrajaka Pitta and weaken the skin barrier. Prolonged chemical and steroid exposure leads to thinning of skin, vascular sensitivity, inflammation, pigmentation, and chronic facial hypersensitivity. Vata causes dryness and fragility while Kapha may produce acneiform eruptions.

Lakshana (Symptoms)

- Facial redness
- Burning sensation
- Thin sensitive skin
- Acne-like eruptions
- Hyperpigmentation
- Dryness and irritation
- Visible blood vessels
- Steroid dependency flare-ups

Ayurvedic Management

1. Shamana Chikitsa (Internal Medicines)

Mahatikta Ghrita

Dosage: 5–10 grams daily
Anupana: Warm milk or water
Duration: 2–3 months

Sarivadyasava

Dosage: 15–20 ml twice daily
Anupana: Equal quantity of water
Duration: 2 months

Guduchi Satva

Dosage: 500 mg twice daily
Anupana: Honey or warm water
Duration: 2–3 months

Gandhak Rasayan

Dosage: 250 mg twice daily
Anupana: Honey
Duration: 2 months

Avipattikar Churna

Dosage: 3–5 grams at bedtime
Anupana: Warm water
Duration: 1–2 months

2. External Therapies

Cooling & Healing Applications

Aloe Vera Gel

Provides soothing and skin barrier repair.

Sandalwood & Yashtimadhu Paste

Useful in burning and redness.

Kumkumadi Taila

Gentle application improves nourishment and complexion.

Coconut Oil Application

Helpful in dry and damaged skin.

3. Panchakarma

Virechana

Best therapy for Pitta-Rakta dominant skin damage.

Nasya

Improves facial nourishment and skin recovery.

Shirodhara

Useful in stress-related facial sensitivity.

Pathya (Wholesome Diet & Lifestyle)

Recommended Foods

- Amla
- Coconut water
- Cow's ghee

- Pomegranate
- Green vegetables
- Fresh fruits
- Mung dal
- Warm water

Healthy Practices

- Use mild herbal skincare
- Avoid unnecessary cosmetics
- Adequate hydration
- Proper sleep
- Stress management
- Gentle cleansing routine

Apathya (To Avoid)

- Topical steroid misuse
- Harsh cosmetic procedures
- Excess makeup
- Spicy and fried foods
- Smoking and alcohol
- Excess sunlight exposure
- Late-night sleeping

Prognosis (Sadhya-Asadhyata)

- Mild cosmetic dermatitis: Sadhya (curable)
- Chronic steroid-damaged skin: Yapya (manageable)
- Early withdrawal of harmful products improves prognosis.

Conclusion

Cosmetic-induced dermatitis and steroid-damaged skin arise due to aggravation of Pitta, Rakta, and damage to Bhrajaka Pitta from prolonged chemical exposure. Ayurveda offers holistic management through cooling therapies, skin rejuvenation, Panchakarma, herbal medicines, dietary correction, and lifestyle regulation. Proper Ayurvedic care helps restore skin barrier function, reduce inflammation, and maintain healthy skin naturally.

Chapter 26

PREMATURE AGING, WRINKLES & SENILE SKIN CHANGES

Introduction

Premature aging, wrinkles, and senile skin changes are characterized by loss of skin elasticity, dryness, fine lines, sagging, pigmentation, and reduced skin vitality occurring earlier than normal aging. In Ayurveda, these changes are primarily associated with aggravation of Vata Dosha, depletion of Rasa Dhatu, Rakta Dhatu, and decline of Ojas. Stress, poor nutrition, excessive sun exposure, and unhealthy lifestyle accelerate skin aging.

Classical Reference (श्लोक)

"वृद्धौ वातप्रकोपः स्यात् त्वचः शोषः प्रभिद्यते ।
वलयः पालितं खालित्यं जरा लक्षणमुच्यते ॥"

— Ayurvedic Classical Reference

Meaning

Aggravation of Vata during aging causes dryness of skin, wrinkles, greying, hair fall, and degenerative changes.

Another reference:

"रसक्षये त्वचो हानिः कान्तिक्षयश्च जायते।"

Meaning: Depletion of Rasa Dhatu leads to loss of skin nourishment and complexion.

Nidana (Causes)

- Aging process
- Excess sun exposure
- Stress and anxiety
- Sleep deprivation
- Smoking and alcohol
- Poor nutrition
- Dehydration
- Excessive cosmetic procedures
- Pollution and environmental toxins

Samprapti (Pathogenesis)

Aggravated Vata causes dryness, loss of elasticity, and degeneration of skin tissues. Depletion of Rasa, Rakta, and Ojas weakens skin nourishment leading to wrinkles, thinning, dullness, and senile changes. Pitta contributes to pigmentation and inflammation.

Lakshana (Symptoms)

- Fine lines and wrinkles
- Dry rough skin
- Sagging skin
- Loss of skin elasticity
- Dull complexion
- Age spots and pigmentation
- Thin fragile skin
- Reduced skin glow

Ayurvedic Management

1. Shamana Chikitsa (Internal Medicines)

Amalaki Rasayana

Dosage: 3–5 grams twice daily
Anupana: Milk
Duration: 3–6 months

Ashwagandha Churna

Dosage: 3–5 grams twice daily
Anupana: Milk
Duration: 3 months

Chyawanprash

Dosage: 1–2 teaspoons daily
Anupana: Milk
Duration: 3–6 months

Brahma Rasayana

Dosage: 1 teaspoon twice daily
Anupana: Milk
Duration: 3 months

Saptamrit Lauha

Dosage: 250 mg twice daily
Anupana: Honey and ghee
Duration: 2 months

2. External Therapies

Rejuvenating Applications

Kumkumadi Taila Massage

Improves complexion and skin elasticity.

Abhyanga with Sesame Oil

Nourishes dry aging skin.

Aloe Vera & Sandalwood Application

Useful in hydration and soothing.

Herbal Steam Therapy

Improves circulation and skin rejuvenation.

3. Panchakarma

Abhyanga

Best therapy for Vata-related aging changes.

Shirodhara

Useful in stress-related premature aging.

Basti

Beneficial in chronic Vata aggravation and tissue depletion.

Rasayana Therapy

Improves tissue regeneration and vitality.

Pathya (Wholesome Diet & Lifestyle)

Recommended Foods

- Amla
- Cow's ghee
- Milk

- Almonds and walnuts
- Fresh fruits
- Green vegetables
- Sesame seeds
- Coconut water

Healthy Practices

- Adequate sleep
- Daily oil massage
- Yoga and meditation
- Proper hydration
- Regular exercise
- Stress management

Apathya (To Avoid)

- Smoking and alcohol
- Excess sun exposure
- Late-night sleeping
- Excess stress and anxiety
- Junk and processed foods
- Harsh cosmetic procedures
- Excess fasting

Prognosis (Sadhya-Asadhyata)

- Mild premature aging: Sadhya (manageable and reversible to some extent)
- Advanced senile skin changes: Yapya (manageable)
- Early Rasayana therapy provides better long-term results.

Conclusion

Premature aging, wrinkles, and senile skin changes arise mainly due to Vata aggravation, tissue depletion, and decline of Ojas affecting skin vitality. Ayurveda offers holistic anti-aging management through Rasayana therapy, Panchakarma, rejuvenating herbs, proper nutrition, and lifestyle regulation. Timely Ayurvedic care helps nourish the skin, improve elasticity, and maintain youthful healthy skin naturally.

Chapter 27

SUN-DAMAGED SKIN & PHOTOAGING

Introduction

Sun-damaged skin and photoaging result from chronic exposure to ultraviolet (UV) radiation leading to pigmentation, wrinkles, dryness, tanning, roughness, and premature aging of the skin. In Ayurveda, these conditions are mainly associated with aggravation of Pitta and Vata affecting Bhrajaka Pitta, Rakta, and Rasa Dhatu. Excessive heat and sun exposure weaken skin vitality and accelerate degeneration.

Classical Reference (श्लोक)

"अतितापेन पित्तं च रक्तं च परिदूष्यते ।
त्वचि दाहो विवर्णत्वं शोषश्चोपजायते ॥"

— Ayurvedic Classical Reference

Meaning

Excess heat aggravates Pitta and Rakta causing burning, discoloration, dryness, and skin damage.

Another reference:

"वातपित्तप्रकोपेन जरा त्वचि प्रवर्तते।"

Meaning: Aggravation of Vata and Pitta accelerates aging changes in the skin.

Nidana (Causes)

- Excess sunlight exposure

- Hot climatic conditions
- Outdoor occupational exposure
- Dehydration
- Lack of skin protection
- Smoking and alcohol
- Poor nutrition
- Stress and sleep deprivation
- Environmental pollution

Samprapti (Pathogenesis)

Aggravated Pitta damages Bhṛajaka Pitta and Rakta leading to tanning, pigmentation, inflammation, and burning sensation. Vata causes dryness, wrinkles, and loss of elasticity. Continuous UV exposure weakens skin nourishment and accelerates photoaging.

Lakshana (Symptoms)

- Tanning and pigmentation
- Dry rough skin
- Wrinkles and fine lines
- Sunburn and redness
- Uneven skin tone
- Loss of elasticity
- Dull complexion
- Premature aging signs

Ayurvedic Management

1. Shamana Chikitsa (Internal Medicines)

Amalaki Rasayana

Dosage: 3–5 grams twice daily
Anupana: Milk
Duration: 3 months

Sarivadyasava

Dosage: 15–20 ml twice daily
Anupana: Equal quantity of water
Duration: 2 months

Mahatikta Ghrita

Dosage: 5–10 grams daily
Anupana: Warm milk or water
Duration: 2 months

Praval Pishti

Dosage: 125–250 mg twice daily
Anupana: Honey or ghee
Duration: 1–2 months

Guduchi Satva

Dosage: 500 mg twice daily
Anupana: Honey or warm water
Duration: 2 months

2. External Therapies

Cooling & Rejuvenating Applications

Sandalwood Paste

Useful in sunburn and burning sensation.

Aloe Vera Gel

Provides cooling and skin repair.

Kumkumadi Taila

Improves complexion and nourishes sun-damaged skin.

Rose Water Compress

Helps soothe inflamed skin.

3. Panchakarma

Virechana

Best therapy for Pitta-dominant photoaging.

Nasya

Improves facial nourishment and complexion.

Abhyanga

Useful in dryness and Vata-related aging changes.

Rasayana Therapy

Supports rejuvenation and skin vitality.

Pathya (Wholesome Diet & Lifestyle)

Recommended Foods

- Amla
- Coconut water
- Cow's ghee
- Cucumber
- Pomegranate
- Fresh fruits
- Green vegetables
- Mung dal

Healthy Practices

- Use natural sun protection
- Adequate hydration
- Avoid midday sun exposure
- Proper sleep
- Yoga and meditation
- Gentle skincare routine

Apathya (To Avoid)

- Excess sunlight exposure
- Spicy and fried foods
- Smoking and alcohol
- Dehydration
- Late-night sleeping
- Excess stress
- Harsh cosmetic procedures

Prognosis (Sadhya-Asadhyata)

- Mild sun damage: Sadhya (curable)
- Chronic photoaging: Yapya (manageable)
- Early preventive care improves long-term skin health.

Conclusion

Sun-damaged skin and photoaging arise due to aggravation of Pitta and Vata causing inflammation, pigmentation, dryness, and premature aging. Ayurveda offers holistic management through cooling therapies, Rasayana treatment, Panchakarma, proper nutrition, and lifestyle correction. Proper Ayurvedic care helps repair sun damage, improve skin vitality, and maintain youthful healthy skin naturally.

Chapter 28

MENOPAUSAL & AGE-RELATED SKIN DISORDERS

Introduction

Menopausal and age-related skin disorders commonly occur due to hormonal decline and progressive tissue degeneration associated with aging. These conditions include dryness, itching, thinning of skin, pigmentation, wrinkles, reduced elasticity, delayed healing, and increased sensitivity. In Ayurveda, menopause and aging are primarily associated with aggravation of Vata Dosha along with depletion of Rasa, Rakta, and Shukra Dhatu leading to loss of skin nourishment and vitality.

Classical Reference (श्लोक)

"वृद्धावस्थासु वातो हि बलवानुपजायते ।
धातूनां क्षयमापन्ने त्वचि शोषो विवर्णता ॥"

— Ayurvedic Classical Reference

Meaning

In advancing age, Vata becomes dominant and depletion of body tissues leads to dryness and discoloration of the skin.

Another reference:

"रसक्षये त्वचा रूक्षा कान्तिहीना च जायते।"

Meaning: Depletion of Rasa Dhatu causes dryness and loss of skin glow.

Nidana (Causes)

- Menopausal hormonal changes
- Aging process
- Nutritional deficiency
- Stress and anxiety
- Sleep deprivation
- Dehydration
- Excess sun exposure
- Smoking and alcohol
- Chronic illness

Samprapti (Pathogenesis)

Aggravated Vata causes dryness, thinning, and degeneration of skin tissues. Decline of Rasa, Rakta, and Shukra Dhatu reduces skin nourishment, elasticity, and moisture. Pitta may contribute to hot flushes and pigmentation, while reduced Ojas weakens skin resilience.

Lakshana (Symptoms)

- Dry rough skin
- Wrinkles and sagging
- Itching and irritation
- Pigmentation changes
- Loss of elasticity
- Thin fragile skin
- Delayed wound healing
- Facial dullness

Ayurvedic Management

1. Shamana Chikitsa (Internal Medicines)

Ashwagandha Churna

Dosage: 3–5 grams twice daily
Anupana: Milk
Duration: 3 months

Shatavari Churna

Dosage: 3–5 grams twice daily
Anupana: Milk
Duration: 3 months

Amalaki Rasayana

Dosage: 3–5 grams twice daily
Anupana: Milk
Duration: 3–6 months

Chyawanprash

Dosage: 1–2 teaspoons daily
Anupana: Milk
Duration: 3 months

Brahma Rasayana

Dosage: 1 teaspoon twice daily
Anupana: Milk
Duration: 2–3 months

2. External Therapies

Rejuvenating Skin Therapies

Kumkumadi Taila Massage

Improves complexion and elasticity.

Sesame Oil Abhyanga

Useful in dryness and Vata disorders.

Aloe Vera Application

Provides hydration and soothing effect.

Sandalwood & Rose Paste

Helpful in cooling and rejuvenation.

3. Panchakarma

Abhyanga

Best therapy for age-related Vata aggravation.

Basti

Useful in chronic Vata-related degeneration.

Shirodhara

Beneficial in stress, insomnia, and menopausal symptoms.

Rasayana Therapy

Improves tissue nourishment and rejuvenation.

Pathya (Wholesome Diet & Lifestyle)

Recommended Foods

- Cow's ghee
- Milk
- Almonds and walnuts
- Sesame seeds
- Amla
- Green vegetables
- Fresh fruits
- Coconut water

Healthy Practices

- Regular oil massage
- Adequate sleep
- Stress management
- Yoga and meditation
- Proper hydration
- Moderate exercise

Apathya (To Avoid)

- Excess fasting
- Dry and spicy foods
- Smoking and alcohol
- Sleep deprivation
- Excess stress and anxiety
- Excess sun exposure
- Junk and processed foods

Prognosis (Sadhya-Asadhyata)

- Mild menopausal skin changes: Sadhya (manageable)
- Advanced age-related degeneration: Yapya (manageable)

- Regular Rasayana and Vata balancing improve quality of life.

Conclusion

Menopausal and age-related skin disorders arise mainly due to Vata aggravation, hormonal decline, and tissue depletion affecting skin nourishment and vitality. Ayurveda offers holistic management through Rasayana therapy, Panchakarma, rejuvenating herbs, proper nutrition, and lifestyle correction. Proper Ayurvedic care helps maintain healthy, nourished, and resilient skin naturally during aging and menopause.

Chapter 29

SKIN BARRIER DYSFUNCTION & DEHYDRATED SKIN DISORDERS

Introduction

Skin barrier dysfunction and dehydrated skin disorders are characterized by dryness, irritation, increased sensitivity, roughness, itching, and impaired protection against environmental factors. Damage to the natural skin barrier leads to excessive water loss and vulnerability to allergens and infections. In Ayurveda, these conditions are mainly associated with aggravation of Vata Dosha along with depletion of Rasa Dhatu and impairment of Bhrajaka Pitta.

Classical Reference (श्लोक)

"वातप्रकोपात् त्वचा रूक्षा खरस्पर्शा विवर्णता ।
रसक्षये त्वचो हानिः स्फुटनं चोपजायते ॥"

— Ayurvedic Classical Reference

Meaning

Aggravated Vata and depletion of Rasa Dhatu produce dryness, roughness, discoloration, and cracking of the skin.

Another reference:

"भ्राजकपित्तदौर्बल्यात् त्वचो रक्षणहानिता।"

Meaning: Weakness of Bhrajaka Pitta impairs the protective function of the skin.

Nidana (Causes)

- Excessive washing and harsh soaps
- Chemical cosmetics
- Cold and dry climate
- Dehydration
- Poor nutrition
- Stress and anxiety
- Sleep deprivation
- Excessive exfoliation
- Aging
- Excess intake of dry foods

Samprapti (Pathogenesis)

Aggravated Vata dries the skin and weakens its protective barrier. Depletion of Rasa Dhatu reduces hydration and nourishment, while impaired Bhrajaka Pitta affects skin metabolism and resilience. Continuous irritation leads to increased sensitivity, itching, and inflammation.

Lakshana (Symptoms)

- Dry rough skin
- Tightness and irritation
- Increased sensitivity
- Flaking and scaling
- Itching
- Cracks and fissures
- Redness
- Dull complexion

Ayurvedic Management

1. Shamana Chikitsa (Internal Medicines)

Mahatikta Ghrita

Dosage: 5–10 grams daily
Anupana: Warm milk or water
Duration: 2–3 months

Ashwagandha Churna

Dosage: 3–5 grams twice daily
Anupana: Milk
Duration: 2–3 months

Amalaki Rasayana

Dosage: 3–5 grams twice daily
Anupana: Milk
Duration: 3 months

Sarivadyasava

Dosage: 15–20 ml twice daily
Anupana: Equal quantity of water
Duration: 2 months

Saptamrit Lauha

Dosage: 250 mg twice daily
Anupana: Honey and ghee
Duration: 2 months

2. External Therapies

Hydrating & Protective Applications

Sesame Oil Abhyanga

Useful in dryness and Vata imbalance.

Coconut Oil Application

Provides hydration and skin barrier support.

Aloe Vera Gel

Helps soothe and repair damaged skin.

Kumkumadi Taila

Improves nourishment and complexion.

3. Panchakarma

Abhyanga

Best therapy for Vata-dominant dehydrated skin.

Basti

Useful in chronic Vata aggravation and tissue dryness.

Shirodhara

Beneficial in stress-related skin sensitivity.

Rasayana Therapy

Improves tissue nourishment and skin resilience.

Pathya (Wholesome Diet & Lifestyle)

Recommended Foods

- Cow's ghee
- Milk
- Almonds and walnuts
- Fresh fruits
- Green vegetables
- Coconut water
- Sesame seeds
- Mung dal

Healthy Practices

- Adequate hydration
- Gentle skincare routine
- Regular oil massage
- Proper sleep
- Stress management
- Avoid over-cleansing

Apathya (To Avoid)

- Harsh soaps and chemicals
- Excess hot water bathing
- Excess fasting
- Dry and spicy foods
- Smoking and alcohol
- Sleep deprivation
- Excessive cosmetic procedures

Prognosis (Sadhya-Asadhyata)

- Mild skin dehydration: Sadhya (curable)
- Chronic barrier dysfunction: Yapya (manageable)
- Early skin barrier restoration prevents chronic sensitivity.

Conclusion

Skin barrier dysfunction and dehydrated skin disorders arise mainly due to Vata aggravation, depletion of Rasa Dhatu, and impaired Bhrajaka Pitta leading to dryness and hypersensitivity. Ayurveda offers holistic management through oleation therapies, Rasayana treatment, Panchakarma, proper nutrition, and lifestyle regulation. Proper Ayurvedic care helps restore hydration, strengthen skin protection, and maintain healthy resilient skin naturally.

Chapter 30

FACIAL PUFFINESS, ROUGHNESS & ENLARGED PORES

Introduction

Facial puffiness, rough skin texture, and enlarged pores are common cosmetic concerns associated with fluid retention, impaired skin elasticity, excessive oil secretion, and poor skin nourishment. In Ayurveda, these conditions are mainly related to Kapha imbalance, Meda Dushti, and impaired circulation along with involvement of Vata and Pitta. Improper diet, stress, lack of sleep, hormonal imbalance, and unhealthy lifestyle commonly aggravate these disorders.

Classical Reference (श्लोक)

"कफमेदोप्रकोपेन गौरवं श्वयथुस्तथा ।
त्वचि स्निग्धत्वरन्ध्रत्वं दोषैः सम्प्रजायते ॥"

— Ayurvedic Classical Reference

Meaning

Aggravation of Kapha and Meda causes heaviness, swelling, oiliness, and enlargement of skin pores.

Another reference:

"वातदोषात् खरत्वं च पित्ताद्रागः प्रजायते।"

Meaning: Vata causes roughness while Pitta contributes to redness and inflammation.

Nidana (Causes)

- Excess oily and salty food
- Sleep deprivation
- Stress and fatigue
- Hormonal imbalance
- Excessive cosmetic use
- Water retention
- Poor digestion
- Sedentary lifestyle
- Pollution and environmental toxins

Samprapti (Pathogenesis)

Aggravated Kapha and Meda cause fluid retention, puffiness, and excessive oil secretion leading to enlarged pores. Vata causes roughness and uneven texture, while Pitta may produce redness and inflammation. Impaired circulation and toxin accumulation further affect skin clarity.

Lakshana (Symptoms)

- Facial swelling and puffiness
- Enlarged open pores
- Rough skin texture
- Oily skin
- Dull complexion
- Mild redness
- Uneven facial appearance
- Skin heaviness

Ayurvedic Management

1. Shamana Chikitsa (Internal Medicines)

Arogyavardhini Vati

Dosage: 250 mg twice daily
Anupana: Lukewarm water
Duration: 2 months

Kaishore Guggulu

Dosage: 1 tablet twice daily
Anupana: Warm water
Duration: 2–3 months

Triphala Churna

Dosage: 3–5 grams at bedtime
Anupana: Warm water
Duration: 2 months

Sarivadyasava

Dosage: 15–20 ml twice daily
Anupana: Equal quantity of water
Duration: 2 months

Gandhak Rasayan

Dosage: 250 mg twice daily
Anupana: Honey
Duration: 2 months

2. External Therapies

Facial Therapies

Multani Mitti & Neem Face Pack

Useful in oily skin and enlarged pores.

Rose Water Compress

Helps refresh and tighten skin.

Kumkumadi Taila Massage

Improves complexion and circulation.

Herbal Steam Therapy

Useful in cleansing pores and improving skin texture.

3. Panchakarma

Virechana

Best for Pitta-Kapha dominant facial skin disorders.

Nasya

Improves facial circulation and skin nourishment.

Udvartana

Useful in Kapha-Meda related puffiness and oiliness.

Pathya (Wholesome Diet & Lifestyle)

Recommended Foods

- Amla
- Green vegetables
- Bitter vegetables
- Mung dal
- Coconut water
- Fresh fruits
- Warm water
- Light digestible food

Healthy Practices

- Adequate sleep
- Facial cleansing routine
- Stress management
- Yoga and exercise
- Proper hydration
- Regular facial massage

Apathya (To Avoid)

- Excess salty and oily foods
- Junk and processed foods
- Excess makeup and cosmetics
- Smoking and alcohol
- Late-night sleeping
- Sedentary lifestyle
- Excess tea and coffee

Prognosis (Sadhya-Asadhyata)

- Mild puffiness and enlarged pores: Sadhya (curable)
- Chronic oily rough skin disorders: Yapya (manageable)
- Lifestyle correction significantly improves skin quality.

Conclusion

Facial puffiness, roughness, and enlarged pores arise due to Kapha-Meda imbalance, impaired circulation, and skin barrier dysfunction. Ayurveda offers holistic management through detoxification, herbal medicines, Panchakarma, proper skincare, and lifestyle regulation. Proper Ayurvedic care helps improve skin texture, reduce puffiness, and maintain healthy radiant skin naturally.

Chapter 31

SKIN TAGS & BENIGN COSMETIC SKIN DISORDERS

Introduction

Skin tags and benign cosmetic skin disorders include harmless growths such as skin tags, small papillomas, benign moles, seborrheic keratosis-like lesions, and localized thickened skin growths. These conditions are generally non-cancerous but may cause cosmetic concern, irritation, or discomfort. In Ayurveda, such growths are associated with vitiation of Kapha, Meda, and Mamsa Dhatu leading to localized tissue overgrowth and obstruction of skin channels.

Classical Reference (श्लोक)

"कफमेदोमांसदुष्ट्या ग्रन्थयः सम्प्रजायते ।
मृदवोऽल्परुजः स्थिराः त्वचि वर्धन्ति देहिनाम् ॥"

— Ayurvedic Classical Reference

Meaning

Vitiation of Kapha, Meda, and Mamsa leads to soft, stable, mildly symptomatic growths over the skin.

Another reference:

"मांसप्रदोषजा ग्रन्थिः शनैर्वृद्धिमुपैति च।"

Meaning: Disorders of Mamsa Dhatu gradually produce localized growths.

Nidana (Causes)

- Obesity
- Hormonal imbalance
- Insulin resistance
- Friction in skin folds
- Excess Kapha-promoting diet
- Sedentary lifestyle
- Genetic tendency
- Aging
- Improper metabolism

Samprapti (Pathogenesis)

Aggravated Kapha and Meda accumulate in localized skin tissues causing abnormal soft growths. Mamsa Dhatu involvement produces tissue proliferation while impaired metabolism and obstruction of microchannels promote persistence of lesions.

Lakshana (Symptoms)

- Small soft skin growths
- Pedunculated lesions
- Cosmetic disfigurement
- Skin-colored or brown lesions
- Friction-related irritation
- Multiple lesions in skin folds
- Slow gradual enlargement

Ayurvedic Management

1. Shamana Chikitsa (Internal Medicines)

Kanchanar Guggulu

Dosage: 1–2 tablets twice daily
Anupana: Warm water
Duration: 2–3 months

Arogyavardhini Vati

Dosage: 250 mg twice daily
Anupana: Lukewarm water
Duration: 2 months

Triphala Guggulu

Dosage: 1 tablet twice daily
Anupana: Warm water
Duration: 2 months

Kaishore Guggulu

Dosage: 1 tablet twice daily
Anupana: Warm water
Duration: 2 months

Triphala Churna

Dosage: 3–5 grams at bedtime
Anupana: Warm water
Duration: 2 months

2. External Therapies

Local Applications

Kshara Karma

Classical Ayurvedic para-surgical procedure useful in removal of skin tags.

Turmeric & Neem Paste

Useful in preventing irritation and inflammation.

Aloe Vera Gel

Provides soothing effect on irritated lesions.

Herbal Cleansing

Maintains hygiene and prevents secondary irritation.

3. Panchakarma

Virechana

Useful in Kapha-Pitta associated skin growth disorders.

Udvartana

Beneficial in obesity and Kapha-Meda imbalance.

Lekhana Therapies

Helpful in reducing excessive Meda accumulation.

Pathya (Wholesome Diet & Lifestyle)

Recommended Foods

- Green vegetables
- Bitter vegetables
- Amla
- Mung dal

- Barley
- Warm water
- Light digestible food
- Fresh fruits

Healthy Practices

- Weight management
- Regular exercise
- Proper hygiene
- Daily yoga
- Adequate hydration
- Maintain healthy metabolism

Apathya (To Avoid)

- Excess sweets and oily foods
- Sedentary lifestyle
- Obesity-promoting diet
- Excess dairy and junk food
- Smoking and alcohol
- Poor hygiene
- Excess daytime sleeping

Prognosis (Sadhya-Asadhyata)

- Small benign skin tags: Sadhya (curable/manageable)
- Multiple recurrent lesions with metabolic disorders: Yapya (manageable)
- Weight control and metabolic correction improve outcomes.

Conclusion

Skin tags and benign cosmetic skin disorders arise due to Kapha, Meda, and Mamsa Dushti causing localized tissue overgrowth. Ayurveda offers holistic management through metabolic correction, herbal medicines, Panchakarma, Kshara Karma, and lifestyle regulation. Proper Ayurvedic care helps reduce recurrence, improve cosmetic appearance, and maintain healthy skin naturally.

Chapter 32

INTEGRATIVE AYURVEDIC COSMETO-DERMATOLOGY

Introduction

Integrative Ayurvedic cosmeto-dermatology combines classical Ayurvedic skin care principles with modern dermatological understanding for maintaining healthy, youthful, radiant skin. It focuses on prevention, rejuvenation, correction of skin imbalance, anti-aging care, and enhancement of natural complexion through internal purification and external nourishment. Ayurveda considers healthy skin as a reflection of balanced Doshas, proper digestion, healthy Rakta Dhatu, and strong Ojas.

Classical Reference (श्लोक)

"समदोषः समाग्निश्च समधातुमलक्रियः ।
प्रसन्नात्मेन्द्रियमना स्वस्थ इत्यभिधीयते ॥"

— Charaka Samhita

Meaning

A person with balanced Doshas, proper digestion, healthy tissues, and pleasant mind and senses is considered healthy.

Another reference:

"वर्णकान्तिप्रदा त्वचा रसायनैः प्रपोष्यते।"

Meaning: Proper rejuvenation therapies nourish the skin and enhance complexion and radiance.

Nidana (Causes of Cosmetic Skin Imbalance)

- Stress and anxiety
- Improper diet
- Sleep deprivation
- Excess cosmetic chemicals
- Pollution and UV exposure
- Hormonal imbalance
- Dehydration
- Poor digestion
- Sedentary lifestyle

Samprapti (Pathogenesis)

Improper lifestyle and Dosha imbalance affect Bhrajaka Pitta, Rakta, Rasa, and Ojas leading to dullness, pigmentation, acne, dryness, premature aging, and reduced skin vitality. Accumulation of Ama and impaired circulation further weaken skin health.

Lakshana (Symptoms)

- Dull complexion
- Acne and pigmentation
- Dryness or oiliness
- Wrinkles and aging signs
- Sensitive skin
- Enlarged pores
- Uneven skin texture
- Reduced skin glow

Ayurvedic Management

1. Shamana Chikitsa (Internal Medicines)

Amalaki Rasayana

Dosage: 3–5 grams twice daily
Anupana: Milk
Duration: 3–6 months

Chyawanprash

Dosage: 1–2 teaspoons daily
Anupana: Milk
Duration: 3 months

Gandhak Rasayan

Dosage: 250 mg twice daily
Anupana: Honey
Duration: 2 months

Sarivadyasava

Dosage: 15–20 ml twice daily
Anupana: Equal quantity of water
Duration: 2 months

Guduchi Satva

Dosage: 500 mg twice daily
Anupana: Honey or warm water
Duration: 2–3 months

2. External Therapies

Cosmetic Ayurvedic Therapies

Kumkumadi Taila Massage

Improves complexion, glow, and skin nourishment.

Herbal Mukhalepa

Using:

- Sandalwood
- Lodhra
- Manjistha
- Turmeric
- Aloe vera

Abhyanga

Daily oil massage improves circulation and skin vitality.

Herbal Steam Therapy

Helps detoxify and rejuvenate facial skin.

3. Panchakarma

Virechana

Best for skin detoxification and complexion improvement.

Nasya

Improves facial nourishment and glow.

Shirodhara

Useful in stress-related skin disorders and rejuvenation.

Rasayana Therapy

Promotes anti-aging and tissue regeneration.

Pathya (Wholesome Diet & Lifestyle)

Recommended Foods

- Amla
- Cow's ghee
- Fresh fruits
- Green vegetables
- Coconut water
- Almonds and walnuts
- Mung dal
- Warm water

Healthy Practices

- Daily skincare routine
- Adequate sleep
- Yoga and meditation
- Proper hydration
- Stress management
- Regular exercise

Apathya (To Avoid)

- Excess cosmetic chemicals
- Smoking and alcohol
- Junk and processed foods
- Excess sun exposure
- Late-night sleeping
- Stress and anxiety
- Excess spicy and fried foods

Prognosis (Sadhya-Asadhyata)

- Cosmetic skin imbalance: Sadhya (curable/manageable)
- Chronic aging and damaged skin: Yapya (manageable)
- Long-term healthy lifestyle provides sustained skin benefits.

Conclusion

Integrative Ayurvedic cosmeto-dermatology emphasizes holistic skin wellness through Dosha balancing, detoxification, rejuvenation, proper nutrition, Panchakarma, and natural skincare. Ayurveda not only improves cosmetic appearance but also enhances overall health and vitality. Proper Ayurvedic care helps maintain naturally radiant, youthful, and healthy skin for long-term wellbeing.

PART 5

LIFESTYLE, HORMONAL & SYSTEMIC SKIN DISORDERS

Chapter 33

HORMONAL & PCOS-ASSOCIATED SKIN DISORDERS

Introduction

Hormonal and PCOS-associated skin disorders commonly include acne, excessive oiliness, pigmentation, hirsutism, scalp hair fall, and darkening of skin folds due to endocrine imbalance and metabolic disturbances. In Ayurveda, these conditions are associated with imbalance of Kapha, Pitta, Vata, Meda Dhatu, and Artava Dushti. Improper diet, sedentary lifestyle, stress, and impaired metabolism contribute significantly to these disorders.

Classical Reference (श्लोक)

"कफमेदोवृतो वायुः स्त्रीणामार्तवदूषणः ।
त्वचि पिडिकाः केशलोपं वर्णदोषं च कारयेत् ॥"

— Ayurvedic Classical Reference

Meaning

Aggravated Kapha and Meda obstruct Vata and disturb female reproductive functions leading to acne, hair fall, and skin discoloration.

Another reference:

"दोषदुष्ट्या त्वचो वर्णः परिवर्तेत् पुनः पुनः।"

Meaning: Vitiated Doshas repeatedly alter skin complexion and texture.

Nidana (Causes)

- PCOS and hormonal imbalance
- Sedentary lifestyle
- Obesity
- Excess sweets and junk food
- Stress and anxiety
- Irregular sleep
- Insulin resistance
- Digestive impairment
- Lack of exercise

Samprapti (Pathogenesis)

Aggravated Kapha and Meda cause hormonal imbalance and blockage of body channels. Pitta vitiates Rakta leading to acne and pigmentation, while Vata disturbance affects hormonal regulation and hair health. Impaired metabolism promotes chronic skin and endocrine disorders.

Lakshana (Symptoms)

- Hormonal acne
- Oily skin
- Facial pigmentation
- Dark neck and underarms
- Excess facial hair
- Hair fall
- Irregular menstruation
- Weight gain

Ayurvedic Management

1. Shamana Chikitsa (Internal Medicines)

Kumaryasava

Dosage: 15–20 ml twice daily after meals
Anupana: Equal quantity of water
Duration: 3 months

Kaishore Guggulu

Dosage: 1–2 tablets twice daily
Anupana: Warm water
Duration: 2–3 months

Chandraprabha Vati

Dosage: 1–2 tablets twice daily
Anupana: Warm water
Duration: 3 months

Arogyavardhini Vati

Dosage: 250 mg twice daily
Anupana: Lukewarm water
Duration: 2 months

Shatavari Churna

Dosage: 3–5 grams twice daily
Anupana: Milk
Duration: 3 months

2. External Therapies

Skin Care Applications

Neem & Turmeric Face Pack

Useful in acne and oily skin.

Kumkumadi Taila

Improves pigmentation and complexion.

Aloe Vera Gel

Helps soothe inflamed skin.

Herbal Cleansing

Useful in reducing excessive oiliness.

3. Panchakarma

Virechana

Best for Pitta-Kapha dominant hormonal skin disorders.

Basti

Useful in Vata-related hormonal imbalance.

Udvartana

Beneficial in obesity and Meda imbalance.

Nasya

Improves hormonal regulation and facial health.

Pathya (Wholesome Diet & Lifestyle)

Recommended Foods

- Amla
- Green vegetables

- Barley
- Mung dal
- Bitter vegetables
- Buttermilk
- Coconut water
- Light digestible food

Healthy Practices

- Daily exercise
- Weight management
- Stress reduction
- Yoga and meditation
- Proper sleep
- Regular menstrual care

Apathya (To Avoid)

- Excess sweets and bakery items
- Junk and fried foods
- Sedentary lifestyle
- Excess dairy products
- Smoking and alcohol
- Late-night sleeping
- Stress and anxiety

Prognosis (Sadhya-Asadhyata)

- Mild hormonal skin disorders: Sadhya (curable/manageable)
- Chronic PCOS-associated disorders: Yapya (manageable)
- Long-term metabolic correction improves outcomes significantly.

Conclusion

Hormonal and PCOS-associated skin disorders arise due to imbalance of Kapha, Pitta, Vata, Meda, and hormonal dysregulation. Ayurveda offers holistic management through metabolic correction, hormonal balancing, Panchakarma, herbal medicines, dietary regulation, and lifestyle modification. Proper Ayurvedic care helps improve skin health, hormonal balance, and overall wellbeing naturally.

Chapter 34

DIGESTIVE-ORIGIN & CONSTIPATION-ASSOCIATED SKIN DISORDERS

Introduction

Digestive-origin and constipation-associated skin disorders arise due to impaired digestion, toxin accumulation (Ama), chronic constipation, and disturbed metabolism leading to acne, dull skin, itching, pigmentation, eczema, and recurrent inflammatory skin conditions. Ayurveda considers digestion (**Agni**) as the foundation of health, and impaired Agni is a major cause of skin diseases through vitiation of Doshas and Rakta Dhatu.

Classical Reference (श्लोक)

"रोगाः सर्वेऽपि मन्दाग्नौ उत्पद्यन्ते न संशयः ।
आमदोषसमुत्थानाः त्वचि विकारकारकाः ॥"

— Charaka Samhita

Meaning

Most diseases arise due to impaired digestive fire and Ama formation, leading to various disorders including skin diseases.

Another reference:

"मलावरोधात् पित्तं च रक्तं च परिदूष्यते।"

Meaning: Constipation and obstruction of wastes vitiate Pitta and Rakta causing skin disorders.

Nidana (Causes)

- Chronic constipation
- Indigestion and weak Agni
- Excess junk and oily foods
- Irregular eating habits
- Excess spicy and sour foods
- Inadequate water intake
- Sedentary lifestyle
- Stress and anxiety
- Suppression of natural urges

Samprapti (Pathogenesis)

Impaired Agni produces Ama which circulates in the body and vitiates Pitta, Kapha, and Rakta. Constipation prevents proper elimination of toxins leading to skin inflammation, dullness, itching, and eruptions. Vata aggravation further disturbs bowel function and skin nourishment.

Lakshana (Symptoms)

- Acne and skin eruptions
- Facial dullness
- Itching and allergies
- Pigmentation
- Constipation
- Coated tongue
- Bloating and indigestion
- Foul body odor

Ayurvedic Management

1. Shamana Chikitsa (Internal Medicines)

Triphala Churna

Dosage: 3–5 grams at bedtime
Anupana: Warm water
Duration: 2–3 months

Avipattikar Churna

Dosage: 3–5 grams at bedtime
Anupana: Warm water
Duration: 2 months

Arogyavardhini Vati

Dosage: 250 mg twice daily
Anupana: Lukewarm water
Duration: 2 months

Gandhak Rasayan

Dosage: 250 mg twice daily
Anupana: Honey
Duration: 2 months

Mahamanjishthadi Kwath

Dosage: 15–20 ml twice daily
Anupana: Equal quantity of water
Duration: 2–3 months

2. External Therapies

Skin Cleansing Therapies

Neem & Turmeric Paste

Useful in inflammatory skin lesions.

Aloe Vera Application

Helps soothe irritated skin.

Triphala Wash

Useful in cleansing and detoxification.

Kumkumadi Taila

Improves complexion and skin nourishment.

3. Panchakarma

Virechana

Best therapy for Pitta-Ama related skin disorders.

Basti

Useful in chronic constipation and Vata imbalance.

Deepana-Pachana Therapy

Improves digestion and reduces Ama.

Pathya (Wholesome Diet & Lifestyle)

Recommended Foods

- Warm water
- Amla
- Green vegetables
- Papaya
- Mung dal
- Buttermilk
- Whole grains

- Fiber-rich foods

Healthy Practices

- Regular bowel habits
- Daily exercise
- Adequate hydration
- Yoga and meditation
- Timely meals
- Proper sleep

Apathya (To Avoid)

- Junk and processed foods
- Excess spicy and fried foods
- Overeating
- Cold and stale foods
- Smoking and alcohol
- Suppression of natural urges
- Sedentary lifestyle

Prognosis (Sadhya-Asadhyata)

- Mild digestive-related skin disorders: Sadhya (curable)
- Chronic constipation with recurrent skin disease: Yapya (manageable)
- Correction of digestion significantly improves skin health.

Conclusion

Digestive-origin and constipation-associated skin disorders arise due to impaired Agni, Ama accumulation, and vitiation of Doshas affecting Rakta and skin tissues. Ayurveda offers holistic management through digestive correction, detoxification, Panchakarma, herbal medicines, dietary regulation, and lifestyle modification. Proper Ayurvedic care helps improve digestion, eliminate toxins, and restore healthy radiant skin naturally.

Chapter 35

NUTRITIONAL DEFICIENCY & METABOLIC TOXICITY SKIN DISORDERS

Introduction

Nutritional deficiency and metabolic toxicity skin disorders occur due to inadequate nourishment, impaired metabolism, toxin accumulation, and deficiency of essential nutrients affecting skin health. These conditions may present with dryness, pigmentation, poor wound healing, acne, dull complexion, dermatitis, brittle nails, and hair fall. In Ayurveda, these disorders are associated with depletion of Rasa, Rakta, Mamsa, and Ojas along with Ama accumulation and Agnimandya (weak digestion).

Classical Reference (श्लोक)

"रसक्षये त्वचा रूक्षा पाण्डुता कान्तिहानिता ।
धातूनां क्षयसम्भूता विकाराः सम्प्रजायते ॥"

— Ayurvedic Classical Reference

Meaning

Depletion of Rasa and body tissues causes dryness, pallor, loss of complexion, and various skin disorders.

Another reference:

"मन्दाग्निना समुत्पन्नो ह्यामो रोगकरः स्मृतः ।"

Meaning: Ama produced due to weak digestion becomes the cause of diseases.

Nidana (Causes)

- Poor nutrition
- Deficiency of vitamins and minerals
- Junk and processed foods
- Chronic digestive impairment
- Metabolic disorders
- Stress and sleep deprivation
- Excess fasting
- Chronic illness
- Smoking and alcohol

Samprapti (Pathogenesis)

Weak digestion impairs proper formation of Rasa and Rakta Dhatu leading to poor skin nourishment. Ama accumulation and metabolic toxins vitiate Doshas and obstruct microchannels causing dullness, pigmentation, acne, and chronic inflammatory skin disorders. Ojas depletion weakens skin vitality and immunity.

Lakshana (Symptoms)

- Dull complexion
- Dry rough skin
- Pigmentation
- Delayed wound healing
- Acne and eruptions
- Brittle nails
- Hair fall
- Fatigue and weakness

Ayurvedic Management

1. Shamana Chikitsa (Internal Medicines)

Amalaki Rasayana

Dosage: 3–5 grams twice daily
Anupana: Milk
Duration: 3 months

Chyawanprash

Dosage: 1–2 teaspoons daily
Anupana: Milk
Duration: 3 months

Ashwagandha Churna

Dosage: 3–5 grams twice daily
Anupana: Milk
Duration: 2–3 months

Guduchi Satva

Dosage: 500 mg twice daily
Anupana: Honey or warm water
Duration: 2 months

Arogyavardhini Vati

Dosage: 250 mg twice daily
Anupana: Lukewarm water
Duration: 2 months

2. External Therapies

Nourishing Skin Therapies

Kumkumadi Taila

Improves complexion and nourishment.

Aloe Vera Gel

Useful in hydration and soothing.

Sandalwood & Manjistha Paste

Helps improve skin tone and inflammation.

Sesame Oil Abhyanga

Provides nourishment and improves circulation.

3. Panchakarma

Virechana

Best for detoxification and Pitta-Ama disorders.

Basti

Useful in chronic tissue depletion and Vata imbalance.

Rasayana Therapy

Improves nutrition, immunity, and tissue regeneration.

Pathya (Wholesome Diet & Lifestyle)

Recommended Foods

- Amla
- Cow's ghee
- Milk
- Almonds and walnuts
- Green vegetables
- Fresh fruits
- Mung dal
- Whole grains

Healthy Practices

- Balanced nutrition
- Regular meals
- Adequate hydration
- Proper sleep
- Yoga and meditation
- Stress management

Apathya (To Avoid)

- Junk and processed foods
- Excess fasting
- Smoking and alcohol
- Sleep deprivation
- Excess spicy and fried foods
- Carbonated drinks
- Sedentary lifestyle

Prognosis (Sadhya-Asadhyata)

- Mild nutritional skin disorders: Sadhya (curable)
- Chronic metabolic toxicity disorders: Yapya (manageable)
- Proper nutrition and detoxification improve long-term skin health.

Conclusion

Nutritional deficiency and metabolic toxicity skin disorders arise due to impaired digestion, tissue depletion, Ama accumulation, and weakened nourishment of skin tissues. Ayurveda offers holistic management through Rasayana therapy, detoxification, Panchakarma, nutritional correction, and lifestyle regulation. Proper Ayurvedic care helps restore skin vitality, improve complexion, and maintain healthy resilient skin naturally.

Chapter 36

STRESS, ANXIETY & SLEEP-DEPRIVATION RELATED SKIN DISORDERS

Introduction

Stress, anxiety, and sleep-deprivation related skin disorders are increasingly common conditions manifesting as acne, eczema flare-ups, psoriasis aggravation, dull skin, dark circles, itching, premature aging, and hair fall. In Ayurveda, mental stress directly affects Vata and Pitta Dosha, disturbs Agni, weakens Ojas, and impairs skin nourishment. Chronic psychological disturbances adversely influence both immunity and skin health.

Classical Reference (श्लोक)

"चिन्ताशोकभयक्रोधैर्वातपित्तं प्रकोप्यते ।
त्वचि दाहं रुजं कण्डूं वर्णहानिं च कारयेत् ॥"

— Ayurvedic Classical Reference

Meaning

Anxiety, grief, fear, and anger aggravate Vata and Pitta leading to burning, pain, itching, and loss of skin complexion.

Another reference:

"निद्रानाशात् क्षयो देहे कान्तिहानिश्च जायते।"

Meaning: Lack of proper sleep causes tissue depletion and loss of skin radiance.

Nidana (Causes)

- Chronic stress and anxiety
- Sleep deprivation
- Emotional disturbances
- Excess mental work
- Irregular lifestyle
- Excess caffeine intake
- Poor diet
- Digital overexposure
- Lack of relaxation

Samprapti (Pathogenesis)

Aggravated Vata disturbs the nervous system and skin nourishment causing dryness, dullness, and premature aging. Pitta aggravation leads to inflammation, acne, redness, and pigmentation. Ojas depletion weakens immunity and skin resilience, increasing susceptibility to chronic skin disorders.

Lakshana (Symptoms)

- Acne flare-ups
- Facial dullness
- Dark circles
- Itching and sensitivity
- Premature wrinkles
- Hair fall
- Dry rough skin
- Disturbed sleep and fatigue

Ayurvedic Management

1. Shamana Chikitsa (Internal Medicines)

Brahmi Vati

Dosage: 1 tablet twice daily
Anupana: Water or milk
Duration: 2–3 months

Ashwagandha Churna

Dosage: 3–5 grams twice daily
Anupana: Milk
Duration: 3 months

Jatamansi Churna

Dosage: 2–3 grams twice daily
Anupana: Warm milk
Duration: 2 months

Amalaki Rasayana

Dosage: 3–5 grams twice daily
Anupana: Milk
Duration: 3 months

Saraswatarishta

Dosage: 15–20 ml twice daily after meals
Anupana: Equal quantity of water
Duration: 2–3 months

2. External Therapies

Relaxing & Rejuvenating Therapies

Kumkumadi Taila Massage

Improves complexion and stress-related dullness.

Aloe Vera Application

Provides soothing and hydration.

Sesame Oil Abhyanga

Useful in Vata aggravation and dryness.

Rose Water Compress

Helps refresh stressed and tired skin.

3. Panchakarma

Shirodhara

Best therapy for stress, anxiety, and sleep disorders.

Abhyanga

Useful in calming Vata and improving circulation.

Nasya

Improves mental relaxation and facial nourishment.

Basti

Beneficial in chronic Vata aggravation and nervous exhaustion.

Pathya (Wholesome Diet & Lifestyle)

Recommended Foods

- Cow's ghee
- Milk

- Almonds and walnuts
- Amla
- Fresh fruits
- Green vegetables
- Coconut water
- Mung dal

Healthy Practices

- Adequate sleep
- Meditation and yoga
- Digital detoxification
- Stress management
- Regular exercise
- Relaxation techniques

Apathya (To Avoid)

- Late-night sleeping
- Excess tea and coffee
- Smoking and alcohol
- Excess screen exposure
- Stress and anger
- Junk and processed foods
- Irregular lifestyle

Prognosis (Sadhya-Asadhyata)

- Mild stress-related skin disorders: Sadhya (curable)
- Chronic psychodermatological disorders: Yapya (manageable)
- Early stress management improves long-term skin and mental health.

Conclusion

Stress, anxiety, and sleep-deprivation related skin disorders arise due to aggravation of Vata and Pitta, impaired Agni, and depletion of Ojas affecting skin and mental wellbeing. Ayurveda offers holistic management through mind-body balancing, Rasayana therapy, Panchakarma, proper nutrition, and lifestyle regulation. Proper Ayurvedic care helps improve skin health, mental calmness, and overall vitality naturally.

Chapter 37

URBAN POLLUTION, SMOKING & ENVIRONMENTAL TOXICITY SKIN DISORDERS

Introduction

Urban pollution, smoking, and environmental toxicity significantly damage skin health leading to premature aging, pigmentation, acne, dullness, allergies, dryness, and chronic inflammation. Continuous exposure to smoke, dust, chemicals, heavy metals, and environmental toxins weakens skin vitality and accelerates degeneration. In Ayurveda, these disorders are associated with aggravation of Pitta, Vata, Rakta Dushti, and accumulation of Ama (toxins).

Classical Reference (श्लोक)

"दूषितवायुसंस्पर्शात् पित्तरक्तप्रदूषणम् ।
त्वचि वर्णक्षयो दाहः शोषश्चोपजायते ॥"

— Ayurvedic Classical Reference

Meaning

Exposure to polluted air vitiates Pitta and Rakta leading to loss of complexion, burning sensation, and dryness of the skin.

Another reference:

"आमविषसमायुक्ता विकाराः कठिनाः स्मृताः।"

Meaning: Disorders associated with toxins and metabolic impurities become chronic and difficult to manage.

Nidana (Causes)

- Air pollution
- Smoking and passive smoking
- Chemical exposure
- Industrial toxins
- Excess UV exposure
- Poor nutrition
- Stress and sleep deprivation
- Excess junk food
- Lack of skin care

Samprapti (Pathogenesis)

Environmental toxins and smoke aggravate Pitta and Rakta causing inflammation, pigmentation, and oxidative damage. Vata causes dryness and premature aging, while Ama accumulation blocks skin channels leading to dullness, acne, and sensitivity. Ojas depletion weakens skin immunity and repair mechanisms.

Lakshana (Symptoms)

- Dull complexion
- Pigmentation and tanning
- Premature wrinkles
- Acne and breakouts
- Dry rough skin
- Allergic skin reactions
- Enlarged pores
- Loss of skin glow

Ayurvedic Management

1. Shamana Chikitsa (Internal Medicines)

Guduchi Satva

Dosage: 500 mg twice daily
Anupana: Honey or warm water
Duration: 2–3 months

Amalaki Rasayana

Dosage: 3–5 grams twice daily
Anupana: Milk
Duration: 3 months

Gandhak Rasayan

Dosage: 250 mg twice daily
Anupana: Honey
Duration: 2 months

Mahamanjishthadi Kwath

Dosage: 15–20 ml twice daily
Anupana: Equal quantity of water
Duration: 2–3 months

Arogyavardhini Vati

Dosage: 250 mg twice daily
Anupana: Lukewarm water
Duration: 2 months

2. External Therapies

Detoxifying & Rejuvenating Therapies

Neem & Sandalwood Face Pack

Useful in pollution-induced inflammation and acne.

Aloe Vera Gel

Provides hydration and skin repair.

Kumkumadi Taila

Improves complexion and skin nourishment.

Herbal Steam Therapy

Helps cleanse skin pores and remove impurities.

3. Panchakarma

Virechana

Best therapy for toxin-induced Pitta-Rakta disorders.

Nasya

Useful in urban pollution exposure and facial health.

Abhyanga

Improves circulation and detoxification.

Rasayana Therapy

Enhances skin vitality and immunity.

Pathya (Wholesome Diet & Lifestyle)

Recommended Foods

- Amla
- Neem preparations
- Coconut water
- Fresh fruits
- Green vegetables
- Cow's ghee
- Mung dal
- Warm water

Healthy Practices

- Regular facial cleansing
- Adequate hydration
- Yoga and pranayama
- Daily exercise
- Stress management
- Use natural skincare products

Apathya (To Avoid)

- Smoking and tobacco
- Excess junk and processed foods
- Excess alcohol
- Sleep deprivation
- Excess sun exposure
- Polluted environments when avoidable
- Harsh chemical cosmetics

Prognosis (Sadhya-Asadhyata)

- Mild pollution-related skin disorders: Sadhya (curable/manageable)
- Chronic toxin-induced skin damage: Yapya (manageable)

- Long-term detoxification and lifestyle correction improve outcomes.

Conclusion

Urban pollution, smoking, and environmental toxicity skin disorders arise due to aggravation of Pitta, Vata, Rakta Dushti, and toxin accumulation causing chronic skin damage and premature aging. Ayurveda offers holistic management through detoxification, antioxidant Rasayana therapy, Panchakarma, proper nutrition, and lifestyle correction. Proper Ayurvedic care helps protect skin, improve resilience, and maintain healthy radiant skin naturally.

Chapter 38

SEASONAL SKIN DISORDERS, HEAT RASHES & PRICKLY HEAT

Introduction

Seasonal skin disorders, heat rashes, and prickly heat commonly occur during hot and humid weather due to excessive sweating, heat exposure, and blockage of sweat channels. These conditions present with itching, redness, burning sensation, tiny eruptions, irritation, and discomfort. In Ayurveda, such disorders are primarily associated with aggravation of Pitta and Kapha along with vitiation of Rakta and Sweda Vaha Srotas.

Classical Reference (श्लोक)

"ग्रीष्मे पित्तं प्रकोपं याति स्वेदवृद्धिः प्रजायते ।
त्वचि दाहकण्डुरागाः पिडिकाश्चोपजायते ॥"

— Ayurvedic Classical Reference

Meaning

During summer season, aggravated Pitta and excessive sweating produce burning, itching, redness, and skin eruptions.

Another reference:

"स्वेदवाहस्रोतसां दोषात् त्वचि विकारसम्भवः।"

Meaning: Disturbance of sweat channels leads to various skin disorders.

Nidana (Causes)

- Excess heat exposure
- Hot and humid climate
- Excessive sweating
- Tight synthetic clothing
- Poor ventilation
- Dehydration
- Spicy and hot foods
- Poor hygiene
- Excess outdoor activity

Samprapti (Pathogenesis)

Aggravated Pitta and Rakta increase body heat and sweating. Kapha along with sweat obstructs skin pores and sweat channels leading to tiny inflammatory eruptions, itching, and burning sensation. Continuous heat exposure worsens irritation and redness.

Lakshana (Symptoms)

- Tiny red eruptions
- Prickling sensation
- Itching and irritation
- Burning sensation
- Excess sweating
- Redness of skin
- Heat intolerance
- Discomfort in body folds

Ayurvedic Management

1. Shamana Chikitsa (Internal Medicines)

Praval Pishti

Dosage: 125–250 mg twice daily
Anupana: Honey or ghee
Duration: 1–2 months

Sarivadyasava

Dosage: 15–20 ml twice daily
Anupana: Equal quantity of water
Duration: 2 months

Guduchi Satva

Dosage: 500 mg twice daily
Anupana: Honey or warm water
Duration: 2 months

Avipattikar Churna

Dosage: 3–5 grams at bedtime
Anupana: Warm water
Duration: 1 month

Amalaki Rasayana

Dosage: 3–5 grams twice daily
Anupana: Milk
Duration: 2 months

2. External Therapies

Cooling Skin Applications

Sandalwood Paste

Useful in burning and prickly heat.

Rose Water Application

Provides cooling and freshness.

Aloe Vera Gel

Helps soothe inflamed skin.

Neem Water Bath

Useful in itching and heat rashes.

3. Panchakarma

Virechana

Best therapy for Pitta-dominant seasonal skin disorders.

Raktamokshana

Useful in severe inflammatory heat-related eruptions.

Takra Dhara

Beneficial in excessive body heat and Pitta aggravation.

Pathya (Wholesome Diet & Lifestyle)

Recommended Foods

- Coconut water
- Amla
- Cucumber
- Watermelon
- Pomegranate

- Buttermilk
- Green vegetables
- Cooling fluids

Healthy Practices

- Wear loose cotton clothes
- Maintain proper hygiene
- Stay hydrated
- Avoid excessive heat exposure
- Regular bathing
- Practice cooling pranayama

Apathya (To Avoid)

- Excess spicy and fried foods
- Direct sunlight exposure
- Tight synthetic clothing
- Smoking and alcohol
- Excess tea and coffee
- Dehydration
- Excess physical exertion in heat

Prognosis (Sadhya-Asadhyata)

- Mild heat rashes: Sadhya (curable)
- Recurrent seasonal skin disorders: Yapya (manageable)
- Seasonal precautions significantly reduce recurrence.

Conclusion

Seasonal skin disorders, heat rashes, and prickly heat arise due to aggravation of Pitta, Rakta, and obstruction of sweat channels during hot weather. Ayurveda offers holistic management through cooling therapies, detoxification, herbal medicines, Panchakarma, dietary regulation, and lifestyle correction. Proper Ayurvedic care helps reduce irritation, maintain skin comfort, and protect skin health naturally during seasonal changes.

Chapter 39

OCCUPATIONAL, HARD WATER & DIGITAL LIFESTYLE SKIN DISORDERS

Introduction

Occupational, hard water, and digital lifestyle skin disorders are increasingly common due to prolonged exposure to chemicals, detergents, polluted environments, excessive screen time, artificial lighting, and mineral-rich hard water. These conditions commonly present with dryness, pigmentation, irritation, premature aging, acne, redness, itching, and skin sensitivity. In Ayurveda, these disorders are associated with aggravation of Vata, Pitta, Kapha, and Rakta Dushti affecting skin integrity and Bhrajaka Pitta.

Classical Reference (श्लोक)

“दूषितस्पर्शसंयोगात् त्वचि दोषप्रकोपनम् ।
रूक्षता दाहकण्डूश्च वर्णहानिश्च जायते ॥”

— Ayurvedic Classical Reference

Meaning

Continuous contact with harmful substances aggravates Doshas in the skin causing dryness, burning, itching, and loss of complexion.

Another reference:

“अतियोगादिन्द्रियाणां विकाराः सम्भवन्ति हि।”

Meaning: Excessive use of sensory organs produces various disorders.

Nidana (Causes)

- Hard water exposure
- Excessive screen time
- Chemical detergents and solvents
- Occupational chemical exposure
- Air-conditioned environments
- Pollution and artificial lighting
- Sleep deprivation
- Stress and mental fatigue
- Excessive cosmetic use

Samprapti (Pathogenesis)

Aggravated Vata causes dryness and premature aging, while Pitta produces redness, pigmentation, and inflammation. Kapha contributes to clogged pores and dullness. Continuous environmental and digital exposure weakens Bhrajaka Pitta and damages the skin barrier causing chronic irritation and sensitivity.

Lakshana (Symptoms)

- Dry rough skin
- Facial dullness
- Pigmentation
- Acne and breakouts
- Skin irritation
- Itching and redness

- Premature wrinkles
- Enlarged pores

Ayurvedic Management

1. Shamana Chikitsa (Internal Medicines)

Amalaki Rasayana

Dosage: 3–5 grams twice daily
Anupana: Milk
Duration: 3 months

Guduchi Satva

Dosage: 500 mg twice daily
Anupana: Honey or warm water
Duration: 2 months

Sarivadyasava

Dosage: 15–20 ml twice daily
Anupana: Equal quantity of water
Duration: 2 months

Gandhak Rasayan

Dosage: 250 mg twice daily
Anupana: Honey
Duration: 2 months

Arogyavardhini Vati

Dosage: 250 mg twice daily
Anupana: Lukewarm water
Duration: 2 months

2. External Therapies

Protective & Rejuvenating Therapies

Aloe Vera Gel

Useful in dryness and irritation.

Kumkumadi Taila

Improves complexion and nourishment.

Neem & Sandalwood Paste

Helps reduce inflammation and pollution-induced damage.

Sesame Oil Abhyanga

Useful in Vata-related dryness and roughness.

3. Panchakarma

Nasya

Best for urban and digital exposure-related facial disorders.

Virechana

Useful in Pitta-Rakta dominant skin irritation.

Abhyanga

Improves skin nourishment and circulation.

Shirodhara

Beneficial in stress and digital fatigue.

Pathya (Wholesome Diet & Lifestyle)

Recommended Foods

- Amla
- Coconut water
- Fresh fruits
- Green vegetables
- Cow's ghee
- Almonds and walnuts
- Mung dal
- Warm water

Healthy Practices

- Limit screen exposure
- Use soft water when possible
- Maintain workplace hygiene
- Regular facial cleansing
- Adequate sleep
- Stress management

Apathya (To Avoid)

- Excess screen time
- Harsh detergents and chemicals
- Smoking and alcohol
- Late-night sleeping
- Junk and processed foods
- Excess cosmetic procedures
- Dehydration

Prognosis (Sadhya-Asadhyata)

- Mild occupational skin disorders: Sadhya (curable/manageable)

- Chronic exposure-related skin damage: Yapya (manageable)
- Preventive care and environmental protection improve outcomes.

Conclusion

Occupational, hard water, and digital lifestyle skin disorders arise due to environmental exposure, Vata-Pitta aggravation, and weakening of the skin barrier. Ayurveda offers holistic management through detoxification, Rasayana therapy, Panchakarma, skin nourishment, and lifestyle correction. Proper Ayurvedic care helps protect skin health, reduce environmental damage, and maintain healthy radiant skin naturally.

Chapter 40

CHRONIC WOUND HEALING, LOW IMMUNITY & NEURO-ENDOCRINE SKIN DISORDERS

Introduction

Chronic wound healing disorders, low immunity, and neuro-endocrine related skin disorders include delayed wound healing, recurrent infections, stress-induced dermatoses, diabetic skin complications, and immune-related inflammatory conditions. These disorders occur due to impaired tissue repair, weakened immunity, hormonal imbalance, chronic stress, and metabolic dysfunction. In Ayurveda, they are associated with Tridosha imbalance, especially Vata and Pitta, Rakta Dushti, Ojas Kshaya, and impaired Dhatu nourishment.

Classical Reference (श्लोक)

"ओजः क्षये शरीरस्य बलहानिर्व्याधिक्षमः ।
व्रणाः कृच्छ्रेण रोहन्ति दोषदुष्टे विशेषतः ॥"

— Ayurvedic Classical Reference

Meaning

When Ojas is depleted, immunity weakens and wounds heal with difficulty due to vitiated Doshas.

Another reference:

"वातपित्तप्रकोपेन व्रणो दीर्घानुबन्धकः।"

Meaning: Aggravation of Vata and Pitta causes chronic and delayed-healing wounds.

Nidana (Causes)

- Diabetes mellitus
- Chronic stress and anxiety
- Hormonal imbalance
- Poor immunity
- Nutritional deficiency
- Chronic infections
- Sleep deprivation
- Smoking and alcohol
- Poor wound care
- Aging and tissue depletion

Samprapti (Pathogenesis)

Aggravated Vata impairs tissue regeneration and circulation, while Pitta causes inflammation and delayed healing. Rakta Dushti and Ama accumulation impair skin repair mechanisms. Ojas depletion weakens immunity leading to recurrent infections and chronic skin disorders.

Lakshana (Symptoms)

- Delayed wound healing
- Recurrent skin infections
- Chronic ulcers
- Weak and fragile skin
- Inflammation and redness
- Discharge from wounds
- Fatigue and low immunity
- Stress-aggravated skin symptoms

Ayurvedic Management

1. Shamana Chikitsa (Internal Medicines)

Guduchi Satva

Dosage: 500 mg twice daily
Anupana: Honey or warm water
Duration: 3 months

Chyawanprash

Dosage: 1–2 teaspoons daily
Anupana: Milk
Duration: 3 months

Ashwagandha Churna

Dosage: 3–5 grams twice daily
Anupana: Milk
Duration: 3 months

Kaishore Guggulu

Dosage: 1–2 tablets twice daily
Anupana: Warm water
Duration: 2–3 months

Gandhak Rasayan

Dosage: 250 mg twice daily
Anupana: Honey
Duration: 2 months

2. External Therapies

Wound Healing Applications

Jatyadi Taila

Useful in chronic wounds and ulcers.

Panchavalkala Wash

Helps cleanse and heal wounds.

Neem & Turmeric Paste

Useful in infection and inflammation.

Aloe Vera Application

Provides soothing and tissue repair support.

3. Panchakarma

Virechana

Best for chronic inflammatory and Pitta-Rakta disorders.

Basti

Useful in Vata-related tissue degeneration.

Rasayana Therapy

Improves immunity and tissue regeneration.

Abhyanga

Enhances circulation and nourishment.

Pathya (Wholesome Diet & Lifestyle)

Recommended Foods

- Amla
- Cow's ghee
- Milk
- Almonds and walnuts
- Green vegetables
- Fresh fruits
- Mung dal
- Coconut water

Healthy Practices

- Proper wound hygiene
- Stress management
- Adequate sleep
- Regular exercise
- Yoga and meditation
- Blood sugar control

Apathya (To Avoid)

- Smoking and alcohol
- Junk and processed foods
- Excess stress and anxiety
- Sleep deprivation
- Poor wound care
- Excess spicy and fried foods
- Sedentary lifestyle

Prognosis (Sadhya-Asadhyata)

- Mild chronic wounds and low immunity disorders: Krichra Sadhya (difficult but curable)

- Severe neuro-endocrine and immune-related disorders: Yapya (manageable)
- Early immune support and wound care improve prognosis significantly.

Conclusion

Chronic wound healing disorders, low immunity, and neuro-endocrine skin disorders arise due to Tridosha imbalance, impaired tissue repair, Rakta Dushti, and Ojas depletion. Ayurveda offers holistic management through Rasayana therapy, Panchakarma, immune strengthening, wound healing herbs, dietary correction, and lifestyle regulation. Proper Ayurvedic care helps improve healing, strengthen immunity, and maintain healthy resilient skin naturally.

PART 6

DOSHA-BASED DERMATOLOGY

Chapter 41

VATAJA SKIN DISORDERS

Introduction

Vataja skin disorders are characterized by dryness, roughness, scaling, cracking, discoloration, pricking pain, and premature aging due to aggravation of Vata Dosha. These disorders commonly occur due to excessive dryness, stress, anxiety, improper diet, aging, sleep deprivation, and tissue depletion. In Ayurveda, Vata affects Twak (skin), Rasa Dhatu, and Rakta Dhatu leading to impaired nourishment and degeneration of skin tissues.

Classical Reference (श्लोक)

"रूक्षः शीतो लघुः सूक्ष्मो चलो खरश्च वायुः ।
त्वचि शोषं खरत्वं च स्फुटनं जनयत्यसौ ॥"

— Ayurvedic Classical Reference

Meaning

Vata, being dry, cold, rough, and subtle in nature, produces dryness, roughness, and cracking in the skin.

Another reference:

"वातप्रकोपात् त्वचा कृष्णा रूक्षा परुषा भवेत्।"

Meaning: Aggravated Vata causes dark, dry, and rough skin.

Nidana (Causes)

- Excess fasting
- Dry and cold food
- Stress and anxiety
- Sleep deprivation
- Aging
- Excessive travel
- Dehydration
- Excessive exposure to cold wind
- Tissue depletion and weakness

Samprapti (Pathogenesis)

Aggravated Vata dries the skin and depletes Rasa and Rakta Dhatu causing roughness, cracking, scaling, and loss of elasticity. Poor circulation and tissue nourishment further aggravate degenerative skin changes and sensitivity.

Lakshana (Symptoms)

- Dry rough skin
- Scaling and flaking
- Cracking and fissures
- Dark discoloration
- Itching
- Pricking pain
- Premature wrinkles
- Thin fragile skin

Ayurvedic Management

1. Shamana Chikitsa (Internal Medicines)

Ashwagandha Churna

Dosage: 3–5 grams twice daily
Anupana: Milk
Duration: 3 months

Mahatikta Ghrita

Dosage: 5–10 grams daily
Anupana: Warm milk
Duration: 2–3 months

Amalaki Rasayana

Dosage: 3–5 grams twice daily
Anupana: Milk
Duration: 3 months

Brahma Rasayana

Dosage: 1 teaspoon twice daily
Anupana: Milk
Duration: 2 months

Saptamrit Lauha

Dosage: 250 mg twice daily
Anupana: Honey and ghee
Duration: 2 months

2. External Therapies

Oleation & Nourishing Therapies

Sesame Oil Abhyanga

Best for Vata-related dryness and roughness.

Kumkumadi Taila

Improves nourishment and complexion.

Aloe Vera Gel

Provides hydration and soothing effect.

Shatadhauta Ghrita

Useful in dry cracked skin.

3. Panchakarma

Abhyanga

Best therapy for Vataja skin disorders.

Basti

Useful in chronic Vata aggravation and tissue depletion.

Shirodhara

Beneficial in stress-related skin disorders.

Rasayana Therapy

Improves tissue regeneration and vitality.

Pathya (Wholesome Diet & Lifestyle)

Recommended Foods

- Cow's ghee
- Milk
- Almonds and walnuts

- Sesame seeds
- Fresh fruits
- Green vegetables
- Mung dal
- Coconut water

Healthy Practices

- Regular oil massage
- Proper sleep
- Stress management
- Yoga and meditation
- Adequate hydration
- Warm food intake

Apathya (To Avoid)

- Excess fasting
- Dry and cold foods
- Excess travel and exertion
- Sleep deprivation
- Smoking and alcohol
- Excess stress and anxiety
- Cold exposure

Prognosis (Sadhya-Asadhyata)

- Mild Vataja skin disorders: Sadhya (curable)
- Chronic degenerative skin disorders: Yapya (manageable)
- Early Vata balancing prevents premature aging and chronic dryness.

Conclusion

Vataja skin disorders arise due to aggravation of Vata Dosha causing dryness, degeneration, roughness, and impaired skin nourishment. Ayurveda offers holistic management through oleation therapies, Rasayana treatment, Panchakarma, nourishing herbs, and lifestyle regulation. Proper Ayurvedic care helps restore hydration, elasticity, and healthy resilient skin naturally.

Chapter 42

PITTAJA SKIN DISORDERS

Introduction

Pittaja skin disorders are characterized by redness, burning sensation, inflammation, rashes, acne, pigmentation, excessive sweating, and hypersensitivity due to aggravation of Pitta Dosha and Rakta Dushti. Excess heat, spicy food, stress, anger, and sun exposure commonly precipitate these conditions. In Ayurveda, Pitta affects Bhrajaka Pitta and Rakta Dhatu leading to inflammatory skin manifestations.

Classical Reference (श्लोक)

"पित्तं दाहकरं तीक्ष्णमुष्णं रक्तप्रदूषकम् ।
त्वचि रागं स्रवं दाहं पिडिकाश्च प्रजायते ॥"

— Ayurvedic Classical Reference

Meaning

Aggravated Pitta causes burning, redness, discharge, inflammation, and eruptions in the skin.

Another reference:

"रक्तदुष्ट्या त्वचि दाहो रागश्चोपजायते।"

Meaning: Vitiated Rakta produces redness and burning in the skin.

Nidana (Causes)

- Excess spicy and sour foods
- Excess heat and sun exposure
- Anger and stress
- Smoking and alcohol
- Excess oily foods
- Sleep deprivation
- Hormonal imbalance
- Hot climate exposure

Samprapti (Pathogenesis)

Aggravated Pitta vitiates Rakta and Bhrajaka Pitta causing inflammation, redness, acne, burning sensation, and pigmentation. Excess heat weakens skin tissues and increases hypersensitivity and inflammatory reactions.

Lakshana (Symptoms)

- Red inflamed skin
- Burning sensation
- Acne and eruptions
- Excess sweating
- Pigmentation
- Itching
- Sensitivity
- Hot flushed skin

Ayurvedic Management

1. Shamana Chikitsa (Internal Medicines)

Sarivadyasava

Dosage: 15–20 ml twice daily
Anupana: Equal quantity of water
Duration: 2 months

Mahamanjishthadi Kwath

Dosage: 15–20 ml twice daily
Anupana: Equal quantity of water
Duration: 3 months

Praval Pishti

Dosage: 125–250 mg twice daily
Anupana: Honey or ghee
Duration: 1–2 months

Guduchi Satva

Dosage: 500 mg twice daily
Anupana: Honey
Duration: 2 months

Avipattikar Churna

Dosage: 3–5 grams at bedtime
Anupana: Warm water
Duration: 1 month

2. External Therapies

Cooling Therapies

Sandalwood Paste

Useful in burning and redness.

Aloe Vera Gel

Provides cooling and healing.

Rose Water Compress

Refreshes inflamed skin.

Kumkumadi Taila

Improves complexion and nourishment.

3. Panchakarma

Virechana

Best therapy for Pittaja skin disorders.

Raktamokshana

Useful in severe inflammatory conditions.

Takra Dhara

Beneficial in excessive Pitta aggravation.

Pathya (Wholesome Diet & Lifestyle)

Recommended Foods

- Amla
- Coconut water
- Cucumber
- Pomegranate

- Buttermilk
- Green vegetables
- Cooling foods
- Fresh fruits

Healthy Practices

- Avoid excessive heat exposure
- Maintain emotional calmness
- Yoga and meditation
- Adequate hydration
- Proper sleep
- Gentle skincare

Apathya (To Avoid)

- Spicy and sour foods
- Smoking and alcohol
- Excess sunlight exposure
- Anger and stress
- Fried foods
- Excess tea and coffee
- Sleep deprivation

Prognosis (Sadhya-Asadhyata)

- Mild Pittaja skin disorders: Sadhya (curable)
- Chronic inflammatory disorders: Yapya (manageable)
- Early Pitta pacification improves prognosis significantly.

Conclusion

Pittaja skin disorders arise due to aggravation of Pitta and Rakta causing inflammation, redness, burning, and pigmentation. Ayurveda offers holistic management through cooling therapies, blood purification, Panchakarma, dietary regulation, and stress management. Proper Ayurvedic care helps calm inflammation and maintain healthy radiant skin naturally.

Chapter 43

KAPHAJA SKIN DISORDERS

Introduction

Kaphaja skin disorders are characterized by excessive oiliness, itching, heaviness, thickening, swelling, sluggish circulation, and cystic lesions due to aggravation of Kapha Dosha and Meda Dhatu. These disorders commonly include oily skin, fungal infections, cystic acne, skin thickening, and sluggish wound healing. In Ayurveda, Kapha affects Twak, Meda, and Lasika causing stagnation and obstruction in skin channels.

Classical Reference (श्लोक)

"कफः स्निग्धो गुरुर्मन्दः स्थिरः शीतो पिच्छिलः ।
त्वचि स्निग्धत्वकण्डूश्च गौरवं जनयत्यसौ ॥"

— Ayurvedic Classical Reference

Meaning

Kapha, being oily, heavy, cold, and stable, causes oiliness, itching, heaviness, and sluggishness in the skin.

Another reference:

"कफमेदोप्रकोपेन त्वचि श्वयथुकण्डुता।"

Meaning: Aggravation of Kapha and Meda produces swelling and itching in the skin.

Nidana (Causes)

- Excess oily and sweet foods
- Sedentary lifestyle
- Excess daytime sleeping
- Obesity
- Poor digestion
- Excess dairy products
- Humid climate
- Lack of exercise

Samprapti (Pathogenesis)

Aggravated Kapha and Meda obstruct skin channels causing excessive oiliness, thickening, itching, cyst formation, and sluggish metabolism. Poor circulation and toxin accumulation promote chronic skin congestion and infections.

Lakshana (Symptoms)

- Oily skin
- Itching
- Thickened skin
- Cystic eruptions
- Swelling and heaviness
- Enlarged pores
- Sticky sweating
- Slow healing

Ayurvedic Management

1. Shamana Chikitsa (Internal Medicines)

Kaishore Guggulu

Dosage: 1–2 tablets twice daily
Anupana: Warm water
Duration: 2–3 months

Arogyavardhini Vati

Dosage: 250 mg twice daily
Anupana: Lukewarm water
Duration: 2 months

Triphala Guggulu

Dosage: 1 tablet twice daily
Anupana: Warm water
Duration: 2 months

Gandhak Rasayan

Dosage: 250 mg twice daily
Anupana: Honey
Duration: 2 months

Nimbadi Churna

Dosage: 3 grams twice daily
Anupana: Warm water
Duration: 2 months

2. External Therapies

Cleansing & Drying Therapies

Neem & Multani Mitti Face Pack

Useful in oily and acne-prone skin.

Triphala Wash

Helps cleanse skin channels.

Nimbadi Taila

Useful in itching and fungal tendency.

Herbal Steam Therapy

Improves pore cleansing and circulation.

3. Panchakarma

Vamana

Best therapy for Kaphaja skin disorders.

Udvartana

Useful in Meda and Kapha accumulation.

Virechana

Beneficial in Kapha-Pitta associated conditions.

Pathya (Wholesome Diet & Lifestyle)

Recommended Foods

- Barley
- Green vegetables
- Bitter vegetables
- Amla
- Warm water
- Mung dal
- Light digestible foods

- Honey

Healthy Practices

- Daily exercise
- Avoid daytime sleeping
- Maintain proper hygiene
- Regular detoxification
- Yoga and pranayama
- Weight management

Apathya (To Avoid)

- Excess sweets and dairy
- Oily and fried foods
- Sedentary lifestyle
- Excess daytime sleep
- Cold heavy foods
- Junk food
- Excess moisture exposure

Prognosis (Sadhya-Asadhyata)

- Mild Kaphaja skin disorders: Sadhya (curable)
- Chronic cystic and thickened skin disorders: Yapya (manageable)
- Proper metabolism correction improves long-term outcomes.

Conclusion

Kaphaja skin disorders arise due to aggravation of Kapha and Meda causing oiliness, itching, thickening, and stagnation in the skin. Ayurveda offers holistic management through detoxification, Kapha-reducing therapies, Panchakarma, herbal medicines, dietary correction, and lifestyle regulation. Proper Ayurvedic care helps restore skin clarity, balance, and healthy function naturally.

BIBLIOGRAPHY

Classical Ayurvedic Texts

1. Charaka Samhita
   Edited with Ayurveda Dipika Commentary by Chakrapani Datta.
2. Sushruta Samhita
   With Nibandha Sangraha Commentary by Dalhana.
3. Ashtanga Hridaya
4. Ashtanga Sangraha
5. Bhavaprakasha
6. Madhava Nidana
7. Sharangadhara Samhita
8. Bhaishajya Ratnavali
9. Yoga Ratnakara
10. Rasa Tarangini

Modern Ayurvedic & Dermatology References

11. Textbook of Dermatology
12. API Textbook of Medicine
13. Davidson's Principles and Practice of Medicine
14. Andrews' Diseases of the Skin
15. IADVL Textbook of Dermatology

Research Journals & Scientific References

16. World Health Organization (WHO) publications on skin diseases and traditional medicine.

17. National Center for Biotechnology Information (NCBI) research articles on dermatology and Ayurveda.

18. Central Council for Research in Ayurvedic Sciences (CCRAS) publications.

19. Peer-reviewed journals on:

- Ayurvedic Dermatology
- Integrative Medicine
- Cosmetology
- Immunology
- Psychodermatology
- Trichology and Skin Sciences

Author's Clinical Experience

20. Clinical observations, case studies, therapeutic protocols, and practical experience of Dr. Mukesh Aggarwal in the field of Ayurvedic dermatology, cosmetology, trichology, and integrative skin care.

www.ingramcontent.com/pod-product-compliance
Lightning Source LLC
LaVergne TN
LVHW022200200926
848481LV00006B/1799
* 9 7 9 8 9 0 5 4 0 4 6 5 8 *